Handbook of

REHABILITATION MEDICINE

Second Edition

Handbook of REHABILITATION MEDICINE

Editors

KONG Keng He
CHUA Sui Geok Karen
THAM Shuen Loong
WONG Chin Jung

Department of Rehabilitation Medicine
Tan Tock Seng Hospital, Singapore

Tan Tock Seng HOSPITAL

World Scientific

Published by

World Scientific Publishing Co. Pte. Ltd.

5 Toh Tuck Link, Singapore 596224

USA office: 27 Warren Street, Suite 401-402, Hackensack, NJ 07601

UK office: 57 Shelton Street, Covent Garden, London WC2H 9HE

British Library Cataloguing-in-Publication Data
A catalogue record for this book is available from the British Library.

HANDBOOK OF REHABILITATION MEDICINE
Second Edition

ISBN 978-981-12-9567-6 (hardcover)
ISBN 978-981-12-9638-3 (paperback)
ISBN 978-981-12-9568-3 (ebook for institutions)
ISBN 978-981-12-9569-0 (ebook for individuals)

For any available supplementary material, please visit
https://www.worldscientific.com/worldscibooks/10.1142/13915#t=suppl

Typeset by Stallion Press
Email: enquiries@stallionpress.com

Printed in Singapore

Preface

The first edition of "Handbook of Rehabilitation Medicine" was published in 2017, and was written with the intent of addressing rehabilitation conditions and scenarios commonly seen in rehabilitation practice in a practical, problem-based manner. The field of Rehabilitation Medicine, like many other fields of medicine, has expanded rapidly over the past 7 years and hence a timely update and curation of the handbook was deemed necessary. Two areas stand out in particular. The first is the role of rehabilitation technology, be it the use of robotics to augment conventional therapy or the use of wearable sensors to allow remote monitoring of a patient's progress. The second is rehabilitation of the 'frail patient' and its accompanying problems of physical deconditioning and sarcopenia. This is of particular relevance given the rapidly ageing population in many countries.

In this second edition, we have also added 2 new chapters. The first is "Sex and sexuality in the disabled", a subject some of readers may not be comfortable to talk about with their patients, or even if they are willing, may not have the skillset to do so. The second is "A holistic approach to return to driving and work after a disability". Depending on the severity of disability, returning back to gainful employment is often a long and arduous journey for many patients, and a dedicated rehabilitation team goes a long way and helping patients achieve this possibility.

We would like to acknowledge the labour of our chapter authors and contributors, without which this second edition would not have been possible. Finally, we would also like to dedicate this handbook to a dear friend and comrade, the late Dr Adela Tow Pei Er who was a stalwart and leading light of the spinal injury programme in our department for many years.

Clinical Associate Professor Kong Keng He
Department of Rehabilitation Medicine, Tan Tock Seng Hospital

Clinical Associate Professor Karen Chua Sui Geok
Department of Rehabilitation Medicine, Tan Tock Seng Hospital

Adjunct Assistant Professor Tham Shuen Loong
Department of Rehabilitation Medicine, Tan Tock Seng Hospital

Adjunct Assistant Professor Wong Chin Jung
Department of Rehabilitation Medicine, Tan Tock Seng Hospital

List of Contributors

CHAN Mei Leng, PhD (Occupational Therapy)
Principal Occupational Therapist
Department of Occupational Therapy

CHAN Wai Lim William, MBBS, FAFRM (RACP)
Senior Consultant, Rehabilitation Medicine

CHUA Sui Geok Karen, MBBS, FRCP
Senior Consultant, Rehabilitation Medicine

HENG Cheryl, BSc (Hons)
Principal Physiotherapist, Department of Physiotherapy

HONG Yun, Bachelor of Health Science (Occupational Therapy)
Principal Occupational Therapist, Rehabilitation Medicine

KIM Jong Moon, MD
Senior Consultant, Rehabilitation Medicine

KONG Keng He, MBBS, MRCP
Senior Consultant, Rehabilitation Medicine

KUAH Christopher, Bachelor of Health Science
(Occupational Therapy), MSc (Neurorehabilitation)
Senior Principal Occupational Therapist, Rehabilitation Medicine

LIM Hui Hui, MSc (Occupational Therapy)
Principal Occupational Therapist
Department of Occupational Therapy

LIM Pang Hung, MSc (Advanced Neuro-Physiotherapy)
Senior Principal Physiotherapist, Rehabilitation Medicine

LOH Yong Joo, MBBS, MRCP
Senior Consultant, Rehabilitation Medicine

List of Contributors

LUI Wen Li, MBBS, MRCP
Consultant, Rehabilitation Medicine

NG Zhi Yen Valerie, MBBS, MRCP
Consultant, Rehabilitation Medicine

ONG Poo Li, MBBS, MRCP
Consultant, Rehabilitation Medicine

PALANIAPPAN K, MBBS, MRCP
Senior Consultant, Rehabilitation Medicine

RATHA KRISHNAN Rathi, MBBS, MPH
Principal Resident Physician, Rehabilitation Medicine

SEE Mei Ting Valerie, Master, Speech Language Pathology
Senior Speech Therapist, Department of Speech Therapy

SENG Wai Ping Alfred, MBBS, MRCP
Consultant, Rehabilitation Medicine

SETIOTA Nuez Odessa, MD
Principal Resident Physician, Rehabilitation Medicine

SOH Yan Ming, Bachelor of Health Science (Occupational Therapy)
Graduate Diploma (Rehabilitation Counselling)
Principal Occupational Therapist, Rehabilitation Medicine

SWAPNA Tony, Bachelor of Physiotherapy
Principal Physiotherapist, Department of Physiotherapy

TAN Ping Ping, MBBS, MRCP
Senior Consultant, Rehabilitation Medicine

TAN Yi Chang Llewellyn, MBBS, MRCP
Senior Resident, Rehabilitation Medicine

List of Contributors

TAY Rong Jie Matthew, MBBS, MRCP
Consultant, Rehabilitation Medicine

TEO Wee Shen, MBBS, MRCP
Consultant, Rehabilitation Medicine

THAM Shuen-Loong, MBBS, MRCP, FAFRM (RACP)
Senior Consultant, Rehabilitation Medicine

TJAN Soon Yin, MBBS, MRCP
Senior Consultant, Rehabilitation Medicine

TOH Ee Mui Shirlene, Diploma Health Science (Occupational Therapy), Master of Health Science (Sexual Health)
Principal Occupational Therapist, Rehabilitation Medicine

WANG Valerie, MPsyClin
Senior Psychologist, Department of Psychology

WEE Seng Kwee, BSc(Hons)(Physiotherapy), PhD (Neurorehabilitation)
Senior Principal Therapist, Rehabilitation Medicine

WONG Chin Jung, MBBS, MRCP
Senior Consultant, Rehabilitation Medicine

YAP Eng Ching, MBBS, MRCP
Senior Consultant, Rehabilitation Medicine

YEN Hwee Ling, MBBS, FRCP
Senior Consultant, Rehabilitation Medicine

*All contributors are from Tan Tock Seng Hospital, Singapore

Contents

Preface v

List of Contributors vii

1 Deconditioning and Prolonged Immobilisation 1

2 Stroke Rehabilitation 17

3 Traumatic Brain Injury Rehabilitation 31

4 Spinal Cord Injury Rehabilitation 51

5 Rehabilitation of the Geriatric Patient 75

6 Cancer Rehabilitation 87

7 Rehabilitation of the Lower Limb Amputee 105

8 Cardiopulmonary Rehabilitation 115

9 Rehabilitation of Chronic Musculoskeletal Pain 125

10 Intensive Care Rehabilitation 149

11 Dysphagia Rehabilitation 165

12 Rehabilitation of Language and Communication Disorders 171

Contents

13 Practical Approach to Management of Spasticity 179

14 Assistive Devices and Orthotics 191

15 Clinical Perspectives on Rehabilitation Technology 213

16 Sex and Sexuality in the Disabled 225

17 A Holistic Approach to Return to Work and Driving After a Disability 235

Index 247

1

Deconditioning and Prolonged Immobilisation

THAM Shuen-Loong, SENG Wai Ping Alfred

Case

Mr Lim, a 69-year-old male with hypertension, diabetes mellitus and bilateral osteoarthritis of the knees, lived alone, and managed his own affairs. He made daily trips to the nearby coffeeshops with the aid of a walking stick and even did weekly marketing at the supermarket, located one bus-stop away.

Mr Lim developed persistent cough and shortness of breath, which were accompanied by high undulating fevers. He was brought to the emergency department, diagnosed with community acquired pneumonia and was promptly admitted.

On the first night of his inpatient stay, Mr Lim decided to walk to the toilet, but unfortunately sustained a minor fall. He was then told to strictly remain in bed and relieved himself with a urinary bottle whenever he felt the need. Eventually, he developed urinary tract infection and incontinence. And he was placed on adult diapers. Subsequently, even though he recovered from his pneumonia and urinary tract infection (UTI), he could not be discharged. He was found to be weaker, and needed assistance for activities of daily living. There was notable deterioration in cognition and mood. He was referred for physiotherapy but had poor motivation to participate. Despite efforts, he could not recover to previous functional levels. Eventually, he was sent to a nursing home as he was not able to manage his own care anymore.

Introduction

As recent as the 1960s, bedrest was commonly prescribed as therapy for a myriad of medical conditions. It was thought to aid in the healing process, thereby hastening recovery time. Even at current, bedrest is often enforced for fear that the mobilising patient might fall. Ironically, efforts to immobilise the patient may cause greater harm than envisioned, leading to increased length of hospital stays and patient disability. Robust evidence accrued over recent years has demonstrated that inactivity and immobility can have negative impacts on body physiology and function.

Deconditioning, immobility, and functional decline

- Deconditioning is defined as a complex series of changes, affecting multiple body systems, following a period of inactivity, immobility, or bedrest
- Functional decline occurs when these bodily alterations lead to a decrement in physical and/or cognitive functioning, and the person is unable to perform tasks such as activities of daily living

Deconditioning can affect people of any age. In the elderly, deconditioning can be more rapid, severe, and often irreversible. Sedentary behaviour is commonly seen in the hospitalised elderly, spending up to 95% of their time or 23 hours in bed or on a chair.

Whilst bedrest may be necessary during stage(s) of certain injuries or diseases, prolonged immobility or bedrest may lead to the detriment of major organs and systems in the human body. These effects are most notably and predictably seen in the musculoskeletal system. Other bodily systems can be affected as well. (Table 1)

Table 1. Complications of immobility.

Body system	Complications
Musculoskeletal system	• Muscle weakness • Muscle atrophy • Contractures • Osteoporosis
Cardiovascular system	• Decreased cardiac output • Reduced resting heart rate • Orthostatic hypotension • Decreased aerobic capacity • Reduced plasma volume • Thromboembolic events (e.g. deep vein thrombosis, pulmonary embolism)
Respiratory system	• Reduced cough & ciliary function • Reduced tidal volume • Reduced vital capacity • Reduced maximum breathing capacity • Reduced functional residual capacity • Increased arterio-venous mismatch • Lowered arterial oxygenation • Increased pneumonia risk

Genitourinary system	• Impaired bladder emptying • Predisposition to stone formation • Urinary tract infection • Incontinence
Gastrointestinal system	• Loss of appetite • Faecal impaction • Constipation • Reduced absorption
Integumentary system	• Pressure ulcers • Dependent edema
Neurosensory system & mood	• Sensory deprivation • Anxiety • Depression • Intellectual/cognitive dysfunction • Sleep disturbance
Metabolic system & mineral balance	• Glucose intolerance • Lowered basal metabolic rate • Increased parathyroid hormone levels • Increased total cholesterol • Altered corticosteroid levels • Increased adrenocorticotropic hormone (ACTH) • Increased serum triiodothyronin (T3) levels • Increased serum calcium levels • Decreased serum sodium levels • Hypercalciuria

Table 2. Early changes during bedrest and immobilisation.

Impact of bedrest in the first 24 hours
• Reduced muscle power by 2–5%
• Reduced circulatory volume by up to 5%
Impact of bedrest in the first 7 days
• Reduced circulatory volume by up to 25%
• Reduced VO_2max by up to 8–15%
• Reduced function residual capacity (FRC) by up to 15–30%
• Reduced muscle strength by up to 5–10%
• Reduced skin integrity
• Reduced self-confidence

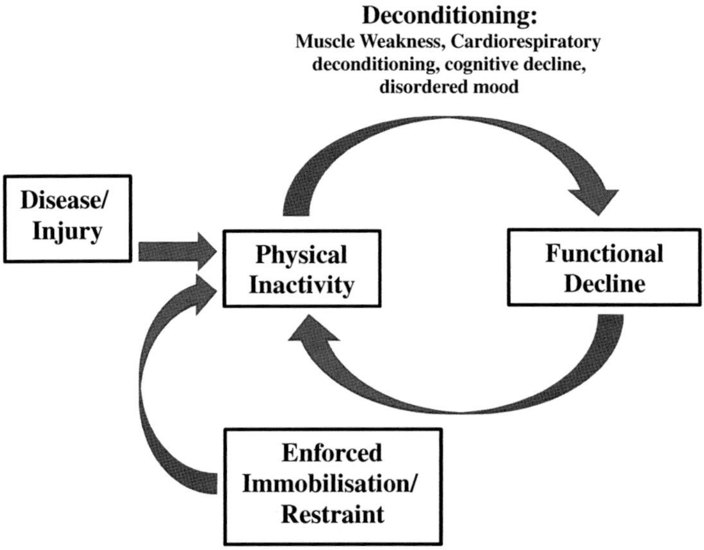

Figure 1. Cycle of functional decline and waning physical activity.

Deconditioning starts in the first day or two of bedrest. The changes in the musculoskeletal and cardiorespiratory systems can impact physical therapy and exercises. Emotional changes can affect motivation, whilst cognitive dysfunction impairs retention and/or carry-over of learnt activities during therapy. As deconditioning sets in, the patient is led into a vicious cycle of functional decline and waning physical activity. (Figure 1)

Body system changes during immobility & recumbency

1. Changes in the musculoskeletal system

Physical changes

a. Muscle
   - Muscle atrophy — reduced muscle mass and fibre size
   - Slow type I muscle fibres are more adversely affected than fast type II muscle fibre loss
   - Muscles of lower limb affected more than upper limbs — primary antigravity muscles (e.g. extensor muscles such as the quadriceps femoris) are most affected

- Affected core muscles, such as the paraspinal and abdominal muscles, lose their tension generating capacity
- Muscle stiffness leads to myogenic contractures if immobilisation is prolonged

The rate of muscle wasting is more pronounced in the first 1–2 weeks of bedrest and slows to a more consistent loss thereafter. It is estimated that an average of 0.5–0.6% total muscle mass is lost per day during bedrest. There is an observed reduction in the number of myofibrils per fibre volume, size and number of mitochondria, muscle fibre nuclei, and a decrease in sarcomeres running in parallel. These findings have been implicated in the loss of muscular strength and endurance in persons with disuse atrophy.

In muscle atrophy, fibres are replaced by fat and connective tissue, and these can be detected with imaging modalities such as magnetic resonance imaging or ultrasonography. Along with muscle fibre atrophy, the synthesis of collagen fibres is also reduced, although this reduction is much less than the reduction in synthesis of muscle proteins. This leads to a relative increase of muscle collagen content and changes its mechano-elastic properties. The muscle stiffness that ensues is further contributed by structural alterations in the muscles, such as changes in the muscle fibre angulations and reduction of sarcomeres in series. When immobilised in a shortened position, that is, extensors in a fully extended position or flexors in a fully flexed position, sarcomere numbers drop, contributing to muscle stiffness and weakness. With muscles held for a prolonged duration in such a shortened state, contractures can develop. Muscles that cross two joints (e.g. gastrocnemius, hamstrings) are particularly prone to immobility-related stiffness and pain.

b. Tendons, ligaments, and cartilage
    - Changes in mechanic-elastic properties, leading to compromised structural function
    - Changes to these structures can be apparent after 4–6 days of immobility and can be attributable to alterations in the collagen fibres leading to joint stiffness and contractures

c. Bone
    - Disuse osteoporosis — bone loss caused by reduced mechanical loading
    - Affects weight-bearing bones more severely than non-weight-bearing ones

- Trabecular and cortical compartments are affected, although some evidence indicates that the loss of trabecular bone occurs earlier and more severely
- Renders affected bone fragile and prone to fracture (i.e. fragility fractures)

Preservation of skeletal mass relies on the mechanical loading applied to the bone by muscle pull as well as the force of gravity. Reduction of mechanical stress on bone inhibits osteoblast-mediated bone formation and accelerates osteoclast-mediated bone resorption leading to reduction of bone mass. It would take a long time for the bone to recover its bone mineral density and strength, much more than the time taken for disuse osteoporosis to set in.

Biochemical/molecular changes

Prolonged immobilisation has been linked to an increased production of various inflammatory mediators, superoxide anions and stress hormone cortisol, which have been purported to be associated with reduced protein synthesis and increased muscle breakdown.

Functional changes and impairment

- Reduced muscular strength
- Decreased endurance and poor work tolerance

During strict bed rest, muscle strength decreases by 1.0–1.5% per day, culminating in about 50% loss from original strength in 5 weeks. The loss of strength is rapid after the first day of immobilisation and reaches its maximum 10 to 14 days later. Maximal instantaneous muscle power ("explosive muscle power") is reduced, and this can be more pronounced than the decrement in the peak muscle strength of one repetitive maximum. With inactivity, reduced motor unit recruitment is observed, as is the reduced ability to activate all motor units during contractions.

For larger and better trained muscles, the faster is the loss of strength and more rapid the rate of deconditioning. Interestingly, the loss of strength and power does not correlate well with the reduction in muscle size and is proportionally more marked.

Metabolic and enzymatic changes in unexercised muscles results from decreased demand for oxygen and reduction in blood supply. On resuming activities, these are quickly depleted, leading to easy fatigability, and poor muscle endurance. The detrimental effects of immobility on the cardiorespiratory system, which result in reduced blood flow and thence oxygen supply to muscle tissues, further compound the problem. Changes in the electrical activity in the muscles and a loss of integrity of the neuromuscular junction potentially also contribute to this early muscle fatiguability.

- ***The weakness and reduced endurance, resulting from inactivity, impair an individual's ability to perform activities of daily living and mobility, jeopardising personal independence***
- ***Pain and stiffness can occur in muscles during periods of immobility, thereby further affecting quality of life***
- ***Chronic immobility and lack of exercise also confer a higher cardiovascular risk***

2. Changes in the cardiovascular system

- Tachycardia — increased resting heart rate; abnormal tachycardic responses on submaximal exercise and on verticalization
- Gradual increase in systolic blood pressure
- Reduced blood volume
- Reduced stroke volume and cardiac output
- Orthostatic/postural hypotension
- Increased risk of thromboembolic events

Stroke volume may decrease by 15% after 2 weeks of bed rest, contributed in part by blood volume reduction and cardiac deconditioning/myocardial thinning. This reduced cardiac output, together with reduced peripheral oxygen utilisation, causes a substantial reduction in maximal oxygen consumption (VO_2max). With prolonged immobility and bedrest, there could be an increase in serum triglycerides and decreases in high-density lipoprotein and apolipoprotein A1. These promote atherosclerosis and increase cardiovascular morbidity.

Owing to an increased peripheral vascular resistance and increased heart rate, there is a gradual increase in systolic blood pressure. The shortened systolic ejection time and diastolic filling time result in a decreased stroke volume. Correspondingly, left ventricular function, cardiac output and overall work capacity are also reduced.

With prolonged recumbency, increased diuresis and progressive decline in blood volume are observed owing to reduced hydrostatic pressure and decreased anti-diuretic hormone release. A reduced circulatory volume of up to 5% and 20% can be seen at 24 hours and 2 weeks respectively, with maximal reduction noted at day 14. As the plasma volume typically decreases more than the red cell mass, blood viscosity increases, leading to the possibility of thromboembolic events.

Orthostatic hypotension can be observed commonly following prolonged recumbency and poses a challenge to activities performed in an upright position. Following recumbency and bedrest, blood from the thorax and abdomen shifts into the legs. Venous pooling in the lower limbs results from impaired vasoconstriction and poor muscle contraction in the legs and abdomen. Coupled with intravascular volume depletion, venous return to the heart is reduced. This results in reduced stroke volume, cardiac output and consequently, a blunted systolic blood pressure response on verticalization. The diminished venous return triggers a rapid heart rate which hampers adequate filling of the right ventricle during end diastole, thereby further compromising stroke volume. The normal sympathetic vasoconstriction response (mediated by norepinephrine, renin, and angiotensin II) is blunted and does little to prevent the drop in blood pressure on verticalization. Consequently, cerebral perfusion may be compromised leading to symptoms of dizziness, fainting, and/or confusion.

Whilst this maladaptive cardiovascular response takes about 3 weeks to be lost in a normal individual, it may set in within mere days in a person with sepsis, major illness/trauma and/or advanced age. The process of restoring normal postural cardiovascular responses can take between 3–10 weeks with remobilisation, and likely even longer for the elderly.

3. Changes in the respiratory system

- Altered pulmonary mechanics — reduced vital capacity, total lung capacity, residual volume, and functional residual capacity
- Ventilation-perfusion mismatch
- Reduced efficacy of cough and secretion clearance
- Increased risk of atelectasis and pneumonia

Recumbency alters lung perfusion and ventilation. Perfusion of blood is gravity dependent and shifts to different parts of the lung in the supine position. The effect of gravity increases venous and hydrostatic pressures in the dependent parts of the lung. Supine positioning also diminishes diaphragmatic movement and restricts chest excursion, leading to shallow breathing and increased respiratory rate. The intercostal and axillary muscles for deep breathing gradually lose their strength and endurance. A change of position from upright to supine results in a reduction of vital capacity (2%), total lung capacity (7%), residual volume (19%), and functional residual capacity (30%). With prolonged recumbency vital capacity and functional reserve capacity may be reduced by as much as 25% to 50%. Ventilation-perfusion mismatch can occur in dependent areas when ventilation is reduced and perfusion increased, leading to arteriovenous shunting with lowered arterial oxygenation.

The effectiveness of coughing is closely related to the functional residual capacity, which is significantly reduced in the supine position. Weakening of the expiratory intercostal and accessory muscles of respiration (especially the abdominal muscles) compromise intrathoracic and intra-abdominal pressure build-up in the compression phase of a cough. Secretions consequently accumulate in the dependent (posterior lobes) parts of the lungs, whilst the anterior regions become dry. This impairs ciliary function and secretion clearance, increasing the risk of atelectasis and pneumonia.

4. Cognitive and affective changes

- Cognitive decline
- Mood alteration (e.g. depression, anxiety)
- Sleep disturbance

Consequent to bedrest and immobility, there could be reduced opportunities for social interaction and mental stimulation. Reduced exposure to social and chronological cues can lead to cognitive, intellectual, and emotional deterioration. Whilst participation in physical activity can enhance cognitive functioning, the effect of reduced physical activity on cognition is less clear.

Prolonged bedrest, together with social isolation, has been found to have greater detrimental effects on these cognitive and affective domains. Cognitive dysfunction in problem-solving and learning ability, psychomotor skills, judgement, concentration, and memory could be affected. Mood issues such as anxiety, depression, irritability, and hostility may be seen. Sleep disturbance and reduced pain threshold can also occur. These can affect the person's motivation, ability to participate in therapy, carry-over of skills and thence functional outcomes. Resumption of ambulation/mobilisation, following prolonged immobilisation can give rise to fear and anxiety (and leading to 'bedrest dependency'), which can further hamper reconditioning efforts.

5. Metabolic and endocrinological changes

- Reduced metabolic rate

Metabolic rate

Basal metabolic rate at 10–24 hours after immobility would have fallen by about 6.9%. And this will continue to fall whilst the body remains sedentary. Increased in adiposity occurs concomitant with a decrease in lean muscle mass. Further weight gain may also be offset by reduced caloric intake (e.g. poor appetite, reduced access to food). As such, body weight may be fairly stable.

Cortisol

Stress hormone cortisol can be released during physical injury, surgery, or even periods of starvation. Hypercortisolemia leads to skeletal muscle breakdown, and this releases amino acids into the bloodstream. Prolonged bedrest also sensitises skeletal muscles to cortisol effects and further worsen sarcopenia.

Calcium

Immobilisation-related hypercalcemia is an uncommon condition, more often seen in patients with spinal cord injury or traumatic brain injury. Disuse causes an increase in bone resorption without concomitant bone production. Hypercalciuria (maximally observed in the 4th or 5th week) in immobility, can occur in tandem with hypercalcemia or even with normokalaemia. This results in total body calcium loss and promotes nephrolithiasis. Even with resumption of physical activity, total calcium loss continues, and negative calcium balance can last for months and even years.

Glucose metabolism and insulin

Prolonged immobilisation and sedentariness have been associated with insulin resistance, impaired glucose tolerance and thence, development of type 2 diabetes. There is a reduced expression of insulin receptors in the skeletal muscle, which desensitises these muscles to the effect of insulin. Hence, a carbohydrate rich meal will result in lower glucose uptake by the muscles and higher blood glucose concentration. Consequently, overproduction of insulin by the pancreatic islets occurs, leading to hyperinsulinemia. Hyperinsulinemia is known to trigger fat deposition and is associated with obesity. Sarcopenic obesity, in which low skeletal muscle mass is coupled with high levels of adiposity, can result.

Management

The various bodily systems, such as the musculoskeletal system and cardiorespiratory system, require constant reinforcement or conditioning to maintain integrity. Pre-emptive interventions can stem deconditioning or, if applied early, mitigate its deleterious effects.

Physical therapy

1. Verticalization

Verticalization often precedes ambulation training in severely deconditioned individuals after prolonged immobilisation. Graduated verticalization, performed with a tilt-table, may be suitable for patients with reduced conscious state or postural intolerance. Active standing can be achieved with person-assistance or equipment (e.g. standing frame). Sitting may be trialled as a form of modified verticalization training (partial body verticalization) for patients intolerant of the standing position.

The importance of early verticalization can be manifold:

a. Mitigate/arrest the cascade of events leading postural hypotension secondary to recumbency

b. Provides axial loading onto the skeletal structures preventing disuse osteoporosis

c. Activates antigravity and postural muscles

d. Improves ventilatory mechanics

e. Promotes normal peristalsis of the intestines and alleviates constipation

f. (Standing) off-loads pressure areas which may otherwise develop into pressure ulcers

Furthermore, verticalization had been noted to stimulate sensorial pathways and postural reactions, which improves the level of arousal and awareness in patients with disorders of consciousness (typically secondary to brain pathologies).

Postural hypotension can limit efforts to verticalize. Non-pharmacological interventions are the foundation of orthostatic hypotension management and can include the following:

a. Bolus water drinking — rapid ingestion of water (500 ml in 2–3 minutes) elicits an increase in blood pressure mediated by the sympathetic nervous system which lasts for 30–40 minutes

b. Compression stockings + abdominal binder

c. Calf compression device

d. Increased fluid intake

e. Increased dietary salt intake (if no contraindication exists) — this may exacerbate hypertension and should be undertaken with caution in hypertensive patients

f. Physical counter-manoeuvres — (e.g. marching on the spot, crossing legs, squatting)

g. Isotonic/isometric strengthening exercises of the lower limb muscles

Pharmacotherapy, such as midodrine (α-adrenergic-receptor agonist) and fludrocortisone (mineralocorticoid agonist), may be trialled for patients who remain symptomatic despite adherence to non-pharmacological interventions.

2. Exercise

Resistance training is essential in combating disuse sarcopenia. A minimum of once a day contraction at 30–50% of maximal strength for 3–5 minutes thrice a week may prevent muscle loss and weakness. Muscle strength improvement can be achieved with the following exercise guide:

a. Concentric or eccentric contraction performed isokinetically or isotonically

b. Intensity of 50–80% of one repetition maximum

c. 8–15 repetition per set, done twice with 1–2 minutes between sets — performed thrice a week

d. Progressive increase in resistance or weights

e. To involve 6 muscle groups (chest, back, shoulder, arms, legs, and calves) — with focus on antigravity muscles, agonist-antagonist muscle groups, and functional training

There has been growing evidence and interest in the use of neuromuscular electrical stimulation to target muscle atrophy. Its effectiveness is, however, limited to the muscle being stimulation and does little for the prevention of total skeletal muscle losses.

VO_2max refers to the maximum amount of oxygen an individual can utilise during maximal exercise and is indicative of a person's cardiovascular fitness and aerobic endurance. The longer the duration of bedrest, the greater the corresponding decline in VO_2max. Daily **endurance training** at 60–80% of VO_2max or at target heart rate is required to maintain or improve aerobic capacity in the deconditioned individual. Resistance exercises performed regularly (3–4 times weekly) for at least 8 weeks can also see improvements in endurance and cardiovascular fitness. It is recommended that at least 150 minutes of moderate intensity (or 75 minutes of high intensity) aerobic activities be performed per week for cardiovascular fitness. Endurance training has been known to improve cardiovascular risk factors (including inflammatory and lipid profile, insulin resistance), reducing the risk of coronary artery disease. Nevertheless, it is recommended that both endurance and resistance training be woven into an exercise regime for maximal benefits. Additional to physical benefits, endurance exercises have purported beneficial effects on cognition (particularly executive functioning) and mood.

Stretching to maintain optimal muscle resting length and viscoelastic properties is critical in maintaining muscle function. Each muscle stretch should be performed at least 2–3 days per week (with daily being most effective). Each muscle group stretch should be held for 10 to 30 seconds, to the point of tightness or slight discomfort (not intense sharp pain). Repeat each stretch 2 to 4 times, amounting to 60 seconds per stretch.

Functional assessment and **task specific training** would be necessary for individuals who may be severely deconditioned (especially coupled with cognitive deterioration) and may be unable to perform activities of daily living.

Even with a high intensity rehabilitation exercise program, the time taken for a full recovery of muscle function can take 2 to 3 times longer than the duration of bedrest or immobility.

Respiratory management

Early verticalization and mobilisation can help to prevent respiratory deterioration. In recumbency, patients should perform regular turning/repositioning, deep breathing, and coughing exercises. Pulmonary hygiene (exercises and procedures that help to clear the airways of mucus and secretions), such as forced expiratory techniques, can also be performed. Chest percussion, postural drainage with oropharyngeal suctioning can prevent aspiration and atelectasis.

Nutrition

Gut changes and reduced appetite are observed in immobilised patients, potentially causing reduced caloric intake and deficient vitamin and minerals. Appropriate nutrition is important for muscle building and works in synergy with exercise. Ranges of 1.2 to 2.0 g/kg (body weight)/day of protein appears to be a reasonable range for muscle building in the deconditioned individual, against a background of replete calories. Up to an additional 0.4 g/kg(body weight)/day of protein would be required to maximise muscle protein synthesis to account for increased anabolic resistance, period of energy deficit and loss due to first pass effect during digestion. Anabolic resistance can be seen in sedentary, obese, and older persons.

Fluid management

Fluid intake and output have to be monitored closely in patients on prolonged bedrest. Judicious replacement of fluid may be necessary due to recumbency-associated diuresis and plasma volume contraction. This can help to mitigate the effects of postural hypotension during verticalization. Patients with poor cognition or who have difficulty accessing fluids may require intervention from the healthcare team (e.g. scheduled fluid intake, intravenous hydration). Fluid supplementation requires careful titration, especially in the elderly, who may concomitantly possess conditions that are sensitive to such adjustments.

Limiting toilet privileges may often also result in a patient self-restricting water intake. Circumventing such barriers (e.g. timed voiding, bedside urinal bottle) may adjunctively help management.

Cognitive stimulation and social engagement

Cognitive stimulating activities help to assuage cognitive decline during prolonged bedrest. Daily orientation by hospital staffing, access to calendars and clocks, can hope to help with patient orientation. Optimisation of sensory inputs (e.g. glasses, hearing-aids) is essential to receive such external cues.

Poor sleep can negatively affect cognition and mood. Sleep hygiene education and enforcement should form part of management regime. Maintenance of circadian rhythm, especially in the hospital, may require environmental modification (e.g. sounds, lights).

Immobilisation and deconditioning can result in altered bodily function and appearance, thereby impacting on the individual's concept of self. Promoting independence, where viable, and engaging the patient in decision-making, shift the locus of control back to the individual, thus fostering self-esteem. Socialisation, achieved with communal activities (e.g. group therapy) and befriending services, can develop the social self. Continued interactions with family and friends are also important to this end. The achieving self can develop with activities such as recreational/diversional, music and pet therapy.

Recommended reading

- Graf C. Functional decline in hospitalized older adults. *Am J Nurs* 2006;106(1):58–67.
- Knight J, Nigam Y *et al.* Effects of bedrest 1: cardiovascular, respiratory and haematological systems. *Nurs Times*. 2009;105(21):16–20.

- Knight J, Nigam Y *et al.* Effects of bedrest 2: gastrointestinal, endocrine, renal, reproductive and nervous systems. *Nurs Times.* 2009;105(22):24–27.
- Kortebein P. Physical inactivity: physiologic impairments and related clinical conditions. In: Frontera WR (ed.) *DeLisa's Physical Medicine and Rehabilitation: Principles and Practice, 6th edition.* Philadelphia: Lippincott Williams & Wilkins (2020), Chap. 38, pp. 873–890.
- Nigam Y, Knight J *et al.* Effects of bedrest 3: musculoskeletal and immune systems, skin and self-perception. *Nurs Times.* 2009;105(23):18–22.
- Wieling W, Kaufmann H *et al.* Diagnosis and treatment of orthostatic hypotension. *Lancet Neurol.* 2022;21(8):735–746.

2
Stroke Rehabilitation

KONG Keng He, YEN Hwee Ling

Introduction

Stroke is the fourth leading cause of death and the leading cause of disability in Singapore. With an aging population, its prevalence is likely to increase. Stroke rehabilitation aims to improve functional outcomes following stroke, therefore reducing the burden of care on society and caregivers, and improving the independence and dignity of the patient.

Common stroke deficits

- **Motor deficits** — at the onset of hemiplegia, arm is often more involved than the leg. Motor recovery in the leg occurs earlier and is more complete than in the arm
- **Sensory impairment**
- **Cognitive disorders** — most common are impairments in attention, memory, and executive functioning
- **Dysphasia** — a language disorder characterised by impaired communication

Table 1. Dysphasia classification.

	Fluency	Comprehension	Repetition	Lesion
Global	Poor	Poor	Poor	MCA, peri-Sylvian region
Expressive (Broca's dysphasia)	Poor	Good	Poor	MCA, frontal
Receptive (Wernicke's dysphasia)	Good	Poor	Poor	MCA, temporal
Transcortical motor	Poor	Good	Good	Frontal
Transcortical sensory	Good	Poor	Good	Temporal
Conduction	Good	Good	Poor	Arcuate fasciculus

*MCA — middle cerebral artery

- **Dysphagia:** defined as difficulty swallowing and may be divided into oropharyngeal or oesophageal dysphagia. Common terminology often used in dysphagia includes:
    - **Laryngeal penetration:** entrance of food in the airway to the level of the true vocal folds
        - Aspiration: passage of food below the level of the true vocal folds
        - Silent aspiration: absence of any outward signs of difficulty during swallowing
    - **Dysarthria:** impairment in articulation of words

Other less common but significant stroke deficits

- **Hemi-neglect:** disorder of attention with failure to report, respond, or orient to sensory stimuli presented to the side contralateral to the stroke. In severe neglect, patients often collide with objects on the affected side, ignoring objects in front of them and attending to only one side of the body. In milder forms of neglect, patients present with various degrees of ignoring the affected side when faced with stimulation on the affected side
- **Apraxia:** disorder of voluntary movement where one cannot execute a purposeful activity despite the presence of adequate mobility, strength, sensation, coordination, and comprehension
    - Ideomotor apraxia: inability to automatically perform a movement and unable to repeat it on command (e.g. unable to walk on command)
    - Ideational apraxia: inability to coordinate individual steps into an integrated sequence (e.g. holds toothbrush but does not bring it to the mouth)
- **Apraxia of speech:** highly variable and unpredictable substitutions of sounds
- **Agnosia:** disorder of recognition that may occur in any of the major sense modalities despite adequate perception in these modalities:
    - Auditory agnosia: unable to match environmental noise with sound source
    - Visual agnosia: unable to identify object on visual confrontation
    - Anosognosia: unaware of loss of an important bodily function, primarily hemiplegia

- **Homonymous hemianopia:** visual field defect involving either the two right or the two left halves of the visual fields of both eyes. It is caused by lesions of the retrochiasmal visual pathways often involving the occipital lobe

Mechanisms of recovery after stroke

- **Neurological recovery**
    - o Resolution of oedema (up to 8 weeks)
    - o Reperfusion of ischaemic penumbra
    - o Resolution of diaschisis
      Diaschisis can be defined as a loss of function within a region distant to the site of the lesion and results from deafferentation of neurons due to the stroke
    - o Neuroplasticity (cortical reorganisation)
- **Functional recovery**
    - o Improvement in activities of daily living and mobility due to recovery of impairment and/or compensation/adaptation
    - o Can continue to improve for some time after neurological recovery is complete

Time course to recovery

- Peak neurological recovery occurs within first 1–3 months
- Recovery continues at a slower pace up to 6 months
- Progress toward recovery may plateau at any stage of recovery

Motor function recovery following stroke

Brunnstrom's stages of motor recovery — describes the evolution of hemiplegia.

I. Flaccidity

II. Some spasticity, basic synergy patterns, minimal movements may be present

III. Increase in spasticity, some voluntary control over synergies

IV. Decrease in spasticity, some selective activation of muscles outside synergy pattern

V. Further decrease in spasticity, most limb movements outside synergy pattern

VI. Disappearance of spasticity, near normal coordination with isolated movements

VII. Normal function restored

Depending on stroke severity and recovery potential, the stages may progress quickly or may be skipped. Generally, hemiplegia with short or absent stage I has better recovery i.e. the longer the stage I, the worse the prognosis; the lower the stage, the poorer the outcome.

Common assessment scales used in stroke rehabilitation

- **Scales assessing impairment**
  - Stroke severity
    - National Institute of Health Stroke Scale (NIHSS)
  - Upper and lower limb
    - Fugl-Meyer Assessment (FMA)
  - Cognition
    - Montreal Cognitive Assessment (MOCA)
  - Balance
    - Berg's Balance Scale
      - Scores from 0 to 56
      - A score of ≥ 41 implies that the person is considered independent and should be able to move around safely without assistance
    - Trunk Impairment Scale (TIS)
  - Depression
    - Hospital Anxiety Depression Scale (HADS)
    - Patient Health Questionnaire-9 (PHQ-9)
- **Scales assessing activity/function**
  - Performance of ADLs
    - Barthel Index/Modified Barthel Index
    - Functional Independence Measure (FIM). The FIM is more comprehensive as it also assesses communication and cognition, which the Barthel Index does not

        - Modified Rankin Scale
            - A global score of disability
            - Scores from 0 (no disability) to 6 (death)
    - Performance of gait
        - 10-metre walk test for assessment of gait speed
            - <0.4 m/s — household ambulator
            - 0.4–0.8 m/s — limited community ambulator
            - >0.8 m/s — community ambulator
        - 6-minute walk test for assessment of aerobic capacity and endurance
- **Scales assessing quality of life**
    - EuroQol-5D (EQ-5D)

Factors influencing rehabilitation outcome

- Intensity of therapy — the axiom "more is better" is generally true
- Task-specificity of therapy
- Early rehabilitation
- Enriched environment

Rehabilitation of the upper limb

Up to half of stroke survivors has residual upper limb weakness and up to one-third will end up with a functionally useless upper limb. Recovery of upper limb function is only as good as recovery of dextrous function, which means the recovery of fine motor movements of the fingers. Apart from conventional therapy, below are some interventions which have been shown to be useful in improving upper limb recovery.

- **Constraint-induced movement therapy (CIMT)**
    - This refers to the forced use of the affected upper limb by restraining the unaffected upper limb to overcome "learned non-use" of the affected limb
    - Involves:
        - Participation in an intensive upper extremity therapy program where the affected upper extremity is used for up to 6 hours per day
        - Restriction of less affected upper limb for up to 90% of waking hours

    - Shaping therapy, a training method in which a motor task is gradually made more difficult as patient gains skills
  - Some degree of motor strength in the wrist and finger extensors is necessary for participation in CIMT

- **Technology-assisted therapy**
  (For more, see chapter on "Clinical Perspectives in Rehabilitation Technology")
  - Use of robotics to enhance therapy intensity

- **Mirror therapy**
  - In mirror therapy, a mirror is placed along the midsagittal plane between the 2 upper limbs, and the patient is encouraged to move the unaffected upper limb while watching its reflection in the mirror, thus providing the illusion that the affected upper limb mirrors the movement of the other limb
  - Mirror therapy allows the activation of mirror neurones involved to stimulate neuroplasticity

Rehabilitation of gait

- Common gait abnormalities:
  - Gait asymmetry: decreased stance phase and prolonged swing phase of the paretic side. Stride length is reduced on the affected side, decreased walking speed, dependence on assistive walking device
  - Hemiplegic gait: hip extension, adduction, and internal rotation, knee extension, ankle plantar flexion and inversion
  - Hip hiking and leg circumduction occur during the swing phase for foot clearance

- **Body weight-supported treadmill training (BWSTT)**
  - Locomotor retraining on treadmill with partial body weight support
  - Enables repetitive practice of complex gait cycles rather than single limb preparatory manoeuvre

- **Robot-assisted therapy**
  (For more, see chapter on "Clinical Perspectives in Rehabilitation Technology")
  - Apart from intensive and repetitive task training, robot-assisted therapy also provides guidance and assistance as needed which can be adjusted as the patient improves

- Robot-assisted therapy used in stroke patients who are unable to walk independently has been shown to result in increases in comfortable walking speed, walking distance, sitting, and standing balance, walking ability and performance in basic activities of daily living, as well as lowering mean heart rate

Rehabilitation of neglect

Interventions for management of neglect include:

- Visual scanning: consistently scan to involved side
- Increasing patient's awareness of or attention to the neglected space
- Compensatory technique focusing on targeting deficits with a specific intervention
    - Use of prisms: optical deviation of visual fields to affected side
    - Eye patching: increase eye movements to contralateral space
    - Hemispatial glasses
    - Arousal strategies: using external sensory stimulus
- Activation strategies: i.e. spatial motor cueing (limb activation and/or application of sensory stimulation)
- Feedback to increase awareness of neglect behaviour involving auditory and visual stimuli

Rehabilitation of dysphasia

(For more, see chapter on "Rehabilitation of Language and Communication Disorders")

Interventions for dysphasia include:

- Behavioural approach
    - Intensive speech and language therapy
    - Melodic intonation therapy
    - Constraint induced aphasia therapy
- Alternative augmentative communication
    - Use of writing, drawing, communication books, electronic communication devices

Rehabilitation of dysphagia after stroke

(For more, see chapter on "Dysphagia in Rehabilitation")

- Instrumental assessment
  - Videoflouroscopy (VFS)/modified barium swallow (gold standard) or FEES (Fibre endoscopic evaluation of swallowing)
- Interventions for dysphagia include:
  - Modification of diet: thickened fluids or modified food textures
  - Enteral feeding for those who are unable to swallow
  - Swallow using manoeuvres such as:
    - Mendelsohn manoeuvre: patient holds the larynx up, either using the muscles of the neck or with the hand, during the swallow, for an extended period of time increasing airway protection
    - Masako manoeuvre: patient protrudes tongue to increase pharyngeal constriction and then swallows
    - Chin tuck: patient flexes the neck before swallow to prevent premature spillage over base of tongue; increasing airway protection by widening the vallecula and putting the epiglottis in a more overhanging position
    - Supraglottic swallow: patient takes a deep breath, holds it and swallows. This adducts the vocal folds and increases the strength of swallowing muscles thus improving airway protection
    - Effortful swallow: patient squeezes all the muscles of swallowing as hard as he can and then swallows
    - Head/neck rotation: patient turns the head/neck to the weaker side, closing off that side and swallows. This directs the food to the stronger side
- Neuromuscular electrical stimulation of muscles of swallowing

Prognostication of recovery after stroke

Importance of accurate prognostication:

- Assist in the decision-making process regarding the allocation of limited and expensive resources
- Enable the setting of appropriate goals during rehabilitation interventions to improve efficacy

- Provide early warnings or triggers for those who fail to recover as predicted
- Provide more specific information to patients and their carers about the expected outcomes

Prognostication of functional recovery

Some of the factors include:

- Age: the elderly (aged over 70 years) tend not to do as well as younger patients
- Initial stroke severity. This is one of the most important prognostic factors. Patients with severe stroke tend to have a poorer prognosis
- Poor functional status on admission to inpatient rehabilitation
- Presence of multiple comorbidities: those suffering from multiple medical conditions tend to have a worse outcome
- Neglect or visuospatial inattention
- Persistent urinary incontinence
- Cognitive impairments

Prognosticating upper limb recovery

PREP2 algorithm (PREP = Predict Recovery Potential)[1]

- This algorithm has been validated for the prediction of outcome of the upper limb as in the first week of stroke onset. It includes the evaluation of:
    - **SAFE score** — a summation of the Medical Research Council (MRC) grading for the strength of Shoulder Abduction and Finger Extension measured within 3 days of stroke onset has been found to be an excellent predictor of recovery of the affected upper limb as well as bimanual hand use. If the score is 8 or more, the patient is predicted to have very good upper limb function after stroke
    - **Age** — age of 80 years has been taken as the cut-off value for consideration in the algorithm
    - **Transcranial magnetic stimulation (TMS)** — is used to test the function of the ipsilesional lateral corticospinal tract projecting to the muscles of the paretic upper limb. Patients in whom TMS is able to elicit motor evoked potentials (MEPs) in the affected upper limb

typically experience greater motor recovery and better outcome than those in whom MEPs cannot be elicited

- For each patient, the PREP2 algorithm predicts one of 4 possible upper limb functional outcomes at 3 months poststroke — excellent, good, limited or none, with a prediction accuracy of 75%.

Prognosticating ambulation

- The most important factor influencing ambulation is the patient's trunk control. Better trunk control increases the odds of independent ambulation
- Trunk control can be assessed in detail using the scale such as the Trunk Impairment Scale or grossly, by assessing the patient's sitting balance. In a retrospective study of 577 stroke patients admitted to our rehabilitation centre, patients with an admission TIS score of 14 or higher had almost a 70% probability of achieving good discharge ambulatory status (defined as being able to walk independently, or at most needing standby supervision)[2]

Common post-stroke complications

- **Shoulder subluxation**
    - Affects up to 80% of stroke survivors
    - Occurs when the shoulder is partially dislocated from the shoulder joint as a result of muscle weakness, especially the supraspinatus and posterior deltoid
    - Can be felt as a gap between the inferior aspect of the acromion and the superior aspect of the humeral head
    - May or may not be associated with hemiplegic shoulder pain
    - Management:
        - Proper handling of the shoulder to prevent further worsening of subluxation. Carers should avoid pulling on the affected arm
        - Taping or strapping of the shoulder may help to realign the shoulder and relieve subluxation-related pain but its long-term effects on reducing subluxation is uncertain
        - Arm slings are commonly prescribed to reduce subluxation, but there is no good evidence of their effectiveness. The common arm sling can encourage flexor synergies, inhibit arm swing, and contribute to contracture development. It can also affect body

image and may discourage the patient from further use of the affected arm

    - Neuromuscular electrical stimulation of the supraspinatus and posterior deltoid is effective in reducing subluxation in the acute and subacute stage of the stroke

- **Hemiplegic shoulder pain (HSP)**
    - Incidence of 5–84% depending on definition of shoulder pain, type, severity, and timing of evaluation
    - Often occurs 2–3 months' post onset of stroke although it can present earlier
    - Leads to impaired upper limb movement, reduced ability to perform ADLs, poor sleep, depression, and worsened quality of life
    - Multiple contributory factors may influence the development of this condition and they can be categorized as follows:
        - Motor factors — significant muscle weakness and muscle tone changes such as spasticity/flaccidity can lead to muscle imbalances around the shoulder joint. The two muscles most often implicated in spasticity-related HSP are subscapularis and pectoralis major which can lead to abnormal scapulohumeral rhythm. Flaccidity of the muscles around the shoulder joint predisposes to glenohumeral subluxation which can result in HSP
        - Soft tissue lesions such as adhesive capsulitis, rotator cuff tendinopathy or tears, bursitis (subacromial, subdeltoid), bicipital tendinopathy
        - Altered peripheral and central nervous system dysfunction — such as somatosensory abnormalities, hemispatial neglect, central post-stroke pain, complex regional pain syndrome, peripheral nerve entrapment, brachial plexus injury
        - The above factors may occur singly or more likely, in combination
    - Management of HSP
        - Prevention of HSP
            - ✓ Early education of patient and caregivers on proper positioning and handling techniques of the affected arm in sitting, lying, and during transfers
            - ✓ Regular ranging of the shoulder and upper limb

      - ✓ Avoidance of excessive pulling and traction on the arm and overhead pulley exercises
    - Analgesics — such as paracetamol, NSAIDS
    - Botulinum toxin injection — treats spasticity involving muscles around the shoulder
    - Corticosteroid injection — intra-articular or subacromial — treats inflammation of bursa and/or rotator cuff
    - Suprascapular nerve block — blocks the nerve which supplies the majority of the sensory innervation to the shoulder joint

- **Post-stroke spasticity**
  - Common complication in the chronic stage of stroke
  - Common patterns of spasticity after stroke:
    - Upper limb — shoulder adduction, elbow flexion, arm pronation, wrist, and finger flexion
    - Lower limb — knee extension, ankle plantarflexion and inversion, toe flexion (claw toes)
    - Can cause pain, contractures and interfere with selfcare and mobility

  (For details, see chapter on "Practical Approach to Management of Spasticity")

- **Post-stroke depression**
  - The commonest psychiatric complication after stroke, with incidence between 11 and 41%
  - Risk factors:
    - History of depression
    - Stroke severity — the more severe the stroke, the higher the risk of post-stroke depression
    - Lesion location — left hemisphere stroke
    - Poor psychosocial support
  - All stroke patients should be screened for depression given its adverse impact on functional outcome
  - Treatment:
    - Psychotherapy
    - Anti-depressants (e.g. selective serotonin reuptake inhibitors (SSRI))

Neuropharmacology in stroke

- **Motor recovery**
  - There are 3 classes of drugs that are sometimes prescribed for facilitating motor and functional recovery after stroke. These are the SSRIs, dopaminergic agents and Neuroaid, a Chinese medicine that is available over the counter. The evidence supporting the effectiveness of these medications is weak
    - A recent Cochrane review showed that the SSRI, fluoxetine did not reduce disability or increase independence after stroke[3]
    - In a large randomized, controlled trial, the dopaminergic agent, L-dopa did not improve walking outcome in stroke patients[4]
    - In The Chinese Medicine Neuroaid Efficacy on Stroke recovery (CHIMES), a randomized, placebo controlled study, Neuroaid was statistically no better than placebo in improving outcome at 3 months when used among patients with acute ischemic stroke of intermediate severity[5]
- **Dysphasia**
  - Medications that have been tried include SSRIs, dopaminergic agents, cholinesterase inhibitors and piracetam. The evidence supporting the effectiveness of these medications is weak[6] (see chapter on "Rehabilitation of Language and Communication Disorders")

Emerging treatment

- **Non-invasive brain stimulation**
  - There are 2 types of non-invasive brain stimulation: repetitive transcranial magnetic stimulation (rTMS) and transcranial direct current stimulation (tdcs)
  - Both rTMS and tdcs work by priming the brain to learn and respond to rehabilitation, and as such, is combined with rehabilitation
  - Both have been explored in post-stroke motor, language, and cognitive recovery, and although the results of some of these studies are encouraging, they are still very much research tools at the present moment
- **Vagus nerve stimulation**
  - Recently, vagus nerve stimulation has been approved by FDA, USA for use in facilitating upper limb recovery after stroke.[7]

References

1. Stinear CM, Winston D *et al.* PREP2: A biomarker-based algorithm for predicting upper limb function after stroke. *Ann Clin Transl Neurol.* 2017;4(11):811–820.

2. Kong KH, Ratha Krishnan R. Truncal impairment after stroke: clinical correlates, outcome and impact on ambulatory and functional outcomes after rehabilitation. *Singapore Med J.* 2021;62(2):87–91.

3. Legg LA, Rudberg A-S *et al.* Selective serotonin reuptake inhibitors (SSRIs) for stroke recovery. *Cochrane Database Syst Rev.* 2021;11(11):CD009286.

4. Ford GA, Bhakta BB *et al.* Safety and efficacy of co-careldopa as an add-on therapy to occupational and physical therapy in patients after stroke (DARS): a randomized, double-blind, placebo-controlled trial. *Lancet Neurol.* 2019;18(6):530–538.

5. Chen LHC, Young SHY *et al.* Chinese medicine neuroaid efficacy on stroke recovery: a double-blind, placebo-controlled, randomized study. *Stroke.* 2013;44(8):2093–2100.

6. Zhang J, Wei R *et al.* Piracetam for aphasia in post-stroke patients: a systematic review and meta-analysis of randomized controlled trials. *CNS Drugs.* 2016;30(7):575–587.

7. Dawson J, Liu CY *et al.* Vagus nerve stimulation paired with rehabilitation for upper limb motor function after ischemic stroke (VNS-REHAB): a randomized, blinded, pivotal, device trial. *Lancet* 2021;397(10284):1545–1553.

3

Traumatic Brain Injury Rehabilitation

CHUA Sui Geok Karen, RATHA KRISHNAN Rathi, WANG Valerie

Introduction

Traumatic brain injury (TBI) is defined as an alteration in brain function, or other evidence of brain pathology, caused by an external force. The alteration in brain function may include:

(i) Any period of loss of consciousness or decreased consciousness, any loss of memory for events immediately before (retrograde amnesia) or after the injury; or

(ii) Neurologic deficits (weakness, loss of balance, change in vision, dyspraxia paresis/plegia, sensory loss, aphasia, etc.); or

(iii) Any alteration in mental state at the time of the injury (confusion, disorientation, slowed thinking, etc.)

External forces causing TBI may include closed or penetrating injuries, acceleration/deceleration movements of the brain without direct head trauma as in the case of battlefield, whiplash, or blast TBI, thus brain imaging (CT brain or MRI diffuse tensor imaging) may confirm neuropathology.

TBI constitutes a considerable portion of the global disability burden and are caused primarily by falls and road accidents and is increasingly recognised as a public health priority.

Adult TBI typically has a bimodal age distribution; in young adults 21–30 years of age, with a male predominance due to road traffic accidents; while a second peak occurs in the elderly >70 years of age, with a female predominance, due to falls.

Classification of TBI

The severity of TBI may be classified as mild, moderate, or severe with reference to the either of the following parameters of loss of consciousness (LOC), initial Glasgow Coma Scale (GCS) score, or duration of post-traumatic amnesia (PTA) (see Table 1).

Table 1. Classification of TBI severity.

Severity	Mild	Moderate	Severe
Structural changes on neuroimaging	Normal	Normal/abnormal	Normal/abnormal
Admission GCS	13–15	9–12	3–8
PTA duration/days	< 24 hours	1–7 days	> 7 days
Neurologic deficits	None	Some deficits and patients often functional	Severe deficits likely

(Legend: LOC: Loss of consciousness, GCS: Glasgow Coma Scale, PTA: Post-traumatic amnesia)

Table for the criteria to stratify the severity of TBI. Contributed by the National Centers for Biotechnology Information.

Post-traumatic amnesia (PTA)

- Characterised by an absence of continuous memory of ongoing events over a 24-hour period and includes the period of coma and anterograde amnesia, often associated with variable periods of confusion, disorientation, and agitation
- Patients are often confused, lacking insight into their deficits, and in need for assistance
- While those in PTA have difficulties laying down new memories on a daily basis, with adverse effects on functional independence, they are able to learn implicitly using procedural memory skills
- A longer duration of PTA, in particular exceeding 4 weeks, correlates with poorer independence levels and vocational integration, and higher institutionalization rates

Clinical and functional assessment of the TBI patient

- An early transfer to a formalised inpatient TBI rehabilitation programme within 6 weeks of admission provides clear benefit in terms of reduced total hospital length of stay, improved functional status, reduced disability, and higher rates of discharge home compared to rehabilitation in acute care settings

Clinical assessment

- Includes history from patient and family for injury details, comorbidities, and socio-demographic factors

- Socio-demographic factors include:
  - Age
  - Gender
  - Race
  - Education years (>12 years denotes improved overall outcomes)
  - Marital status
  - Living situation
  - Socioeconomic factors "(premorbid employment associated with better functional outcomes)"
  - Social supports
- Premorbid diseases (e.g. cardiovascular risk factors, presence of renal failure or active cancers): may require specific precautions in terms of blood pressure, heart rate limits, etc.
- Comorbidities: epilepsy, depression, psychosis, alcoholism, substance abuse, cerebral palsy, learning disorders, as these may need active intervention to prevent secondary TBIs
- For those with concomitant polytrauma, ask for activity or weight bearing or joint range of motion restrictions and their recommended durations
- Perform a detailed physical examination, with particular focus on central and peripheral nervous system, cranial nerve examination, vision, hearing, and somatosensory examination, tone, joint range of motion and pain.
- Serial clinical examinations for inpatient TBI may be required due to poor tolerance from reduced arousal, agitation, poor sleep patterns, or pain which may degrade performance

Outcome scales in TBI from coma to community: main focus

- Glasgow Coma Scale (GCS): initial assessment of TBI severity
- Disability rating scale: conscious level, disability, employability
- Rancho Los Amigos Levels of Cognitive Functioning (10 levels): neuro-behavioural levels
- Modified Barthel Index (0–100): ADL independence levels
- Glasgow Outcome Scale (GOS): global function, vocational, societal roles
- Glasgow Outcome Scale-Extended (GOS-E): expanded global function, vocational, societal roles

- PTA scales: Westmead Post-Traumatic Amnesia scale or Galveston Orientation and Amnesia test
- Montreal Cognitive Assessment — MoCA: brief cognitive screen upon emergence from PTA
- Formal neuropsychological assessment at > 6–12 months post-TBI for objective quantification of neurocognitive deficits and develop an individualised cognitive rehabilitation plan for the future

Prognosis of TBI outcome

- Advanced age is associated with universally poorer outcomes
    - Age >80 years predicts a significantly higher mortality by 4–6 times
    - The age of a severe TBI at presentation is related to the likelihood of death with a critical threshold at the age of 50 years
    - For every 10 years of age, outcome worsens by 40–50%
- GCS scores of 3–5 were associated with poor GOS
- Absent bilateral pupillary responses are associated with high mortality rates
- PTA duration exceeding:
    - 4 weeks associated with poorer return to work
    - 8 weeks associated with poorer return to independent ADL
    - 12 weeks associated with higher functional disability, i.e. assistance needed for basic ADLs
- Brain imaging:
    - CT/MRI findings related to TBI also provide important prognostic information:
        - CT findings of subarachnoid haemorrhage, intraventricular haemorrhage, cisternal effacement, significant midline shift, epidural or subdural haemorrhage (epidural better that subdural) are associated with worse outcomes. Contusions had a modest effect on prognosis
        - Diffuse axonal injury (DAI) on MRI affecting brainstem or corpus callosum had a poorer outcome

- Other factors associated with better outcomes and lower mortality include:
    - Presence of preinjury employment
    - Higher educational levels >12 years
    - Higher socioeconomic status
    - Absence of a history of alcohol and drug abuse

Post-traumatic agitation after TBI: a rehabilitation approach

Definition

- A delirium subtype unique to TBI during period of post-traumatic amnesia (PTA)
- Characterised by combination of physical restlessness, akathisia, verbal disinhibition, emotional lability, and/or aggression (to self, surroundings, or others)

Standardised scales to assess PTA and agitation

- Agitated Behaviour Scale (ABS, 0–56): performed several times a day by rehab team to serially monitor progression and treatment effectiveness. Scores >21 indicate severe agitation, <14 implies nil agitation
- Westmead PTA Scale (WMPTAS): assess severity, duration and progress of PTA
- Rancho Los Amigos-Levels of Cognitive Functioning Scale (RLAS I-X): a neurobehavioral scale to indicate patient's level of cognitive functioning and recommended functional levels/need for assistance
- Confused, agitated patients are RLAS IV level

Management of post-traumatic agitation

- Diagnosis is made clinically: observation or witnessed reports of motor restlessness, verbal disinhibition, emotional lability, or aggression
- Rule out potentially reversible medical, physical, psychiatric causes of delirium:
    - Physical: pain, environmental factors (excessive stimulation from noise, visual stimuli, physical restraints, IV cannula, urinary catheters,

tracheostomy, feeding tubes/lines), unmet physiological needs (thirst, hunger, humidity/heat, bladder/bowel distension, fear, etc.)
  - Medical: metabolic disturbances (hyponatraemia, hypercalcemia, dehydration etc.), infection, hypoxemia, pulmonary embolism, urinary retention, constipation, hydrocephalus, seizures, new intracranial collections
  - Substance/medication related: iatrogenic from psychotropic drug use, alcohol, opioids, nicotine, or substance abuse withdrawal
  - Psychiatric: premorbid psychiatric diagnosis (e.g. psychosis, schizophrenia, etc.), sundowning in patients with dementia

- Laboratory tests: FBC, urea, electrolytes, glucose, calcium, magnesium, phosphate, urine toxicology screen, CT/MRI of brain, EEG
- Mainstay of management is **non-pharmacological**, focusing on serial monitoring, environmental modification, behavioural modification for patient and staff safety, and family education. The second-line management is the **judicious use of neuropharmacological drugs**

Non-pharmacological management includes:

- Environmental and rehabilitation milieu modification:
  - Reduce visual and auditory stimuli: reduce number of visitors, single room if possible, dimmable soft lighting, reduce external corridor lights, avoid continuous stimulation from TV, music, etc.
  - Maintain comfortable room temperature and humidity
  - Restraint-free care, minimise the use of hand, leg, body restraints, minimise lines/tubes/catheters
  - Pad bed rails, netted beds or floor beds for motor restlessness to reduce injury/fall risk
  - Frequent re-orientation by staff/family, consistent therapy schedule and therapists where possible
  - Reduce demands of therapy and goals; allow a flexible approach
  - Therapy in a quiet room with reduced visual/auditory stimulation
  - Environmental familiarisation: allow personal possessions by bedside
  - Regulate sleep-wake cycles
  - Timed toileting/voiding
  - Monitor ABS regularly
  - Daily team huddles

- Behaviour modification by rehabilitation team:
  - Tolerate excessive behaviours if safety is not compromised, allow supervised pacing, wheel patient around ward
  - De-escalation techniques: re direction, non-confrontational speech, speak calmly and slowly, explain prior to procedure, avoid crowding the patient or approaching from the front, positive reinforcement
  - Avoid arguing with patient or accusing patient of bad behaviours
  - Time out on the spot (TOOTS) if patient escalates
  - Protect staff from injury (enter in pairs, remove lanyards, tie up long hair)

Pharmacological: judicious use of evidenced-based neuropharmacology

- Review medications and discontinue those that may worsen agitation before starting new medications e.g.:
  - Opioids
  - Anticholinergics
  - Sedatives and tranquilisers (e.g. benzodiazepines)
- Start low and go slow in titration, watch for adverse side effects (excessive sedation, cognitive impairing side effects)
- Treat pain adequately
- Acute management of acute agitation escalation
  - Haloperidol IM/IV (1–2 mg q6-8H with maximum of 10 mg/24 hour), syrup Haloperidol drops 0.1-0.2mg q6-8H
  - IM/IV lorazepam 2–4 mg stat (0.05 mg/kg/BW) is useful due to rapid onset in 1–3 mins
- Medications
  - Beta blockers
    - Propranolol: best evidence for treating post-TBI agitation, reduces agitation intensity, restlessness
  - Anti-epileptic drugs
    - Valproic acid: mood stabilising, limited adverse effects on cognition, safer side effect profile. Monitor liver function
    - Carbamazepine: mood stabilising, pain relief (ensure HLA-B*1502 genotype negative); Monitor sodium, liver function

  - Antipsychotics
    - Typical anti psychotics: increases PTA duration
    - Short-term use of Haloperidol drops
    - Atypical antipsychotics: Olanzapine and Quetiapine
  - Neurostimulants
    - Methylphenidate: increases attention span, processing speed, reduces cognitive fatigue. Monitor heart rate, blood pressure

- Monitor and regulate sleep-wake cycle
  - Melatonin
  - Tricyclic anti-depressants: Amitriptyline, Nortriptyline (monitor for postural hypotension)
  - SSRI, SNRI with sedative potential: Fluvoxamine, Mirtazapine
  - Atypical Benzodiazepines: Zopiclone, Zolpidem (these can impair attention and memory)
  - Avoid use of Benzodiazepines unless patient is a premorbid chronic user

Management of specific post-TBI complications

1. Paroxysmal sympathetic hyperactivity (PSH)

Definition

- PSH is a disorder of autonomic function, characterised by paroxysmal episodes of sympathetic activity
- Onset is rapid for tachycardia, hypertension, tachypnoea, fever, sweating, spasticity with dystonia
- Diagnosis is clinical. Investigations are needed to exclude secondary sepsis, pulmonary embolism, seizures, etc.
- Peak prevalence: 9 to 13 days post-TBI
- Associated with moderate to severe TBI, DAI, intraventricular haemorrhage, subarachnoid haemorrhage, hypoxic ischemic injury, secondary hydrocephalus

Undiagnosed or untreated PSH can result in increased mortality and inappropriate management (excessive investigations or unnecessary antibiotics)

Management

- Identify triggers and avoid them (e.g. loud sounds, alarms, urinary retention, suctioning)
- Ensure adequate hydration, electrolyte replacement, cooling and caloric intake to counter increased metabolic demands
- Pharmacological
  - Abortive: IV Morphine, Propofol, Benzodiazepines, Clonidine
  - Preventive: oral: Propranolol, Clonidine, Baclofen, Gabapentin, Morphine, Benzodiazepines

Prognosis

- Most cases resolve in a year, however a prolonged subclinical state may persist
- PSH is associated with worse long-term functional outcomes, longer hospitalisation, and higher mortality

2. Post-traumatic seizures

- Post-traumatic seizure (PTS) is an initial or recurrent seizure episode (post-traumatic epilepsy-PTE) not attributable to another obvious cause after a TBI
- 5 to 7% of hospitalised TBI patients have PTS
- Risk of PTS is highest in the first two years after TBI
- PTS is classified into **early PTS**: within 7 days of TBI or **late PTS**: after 7 days of TBI

Risk factors for PTS

- Type of patient: older, chronic alcohol use, past history of seizures/epilepsy
- Type of injury: penetrating TBI (e.g. gunshot wounds, depressed skull fractures, focal contusions, focal neurological deficit, severe TBI, intracranial, surgery)
- 25% of patients with early PTS will develop PTE, whereas 86% of patients with late PTS will develop PTE

Prophylactic treatment for seizures

- Moderate to severe TBI with increased risk for PTS are treated with prophylactic anti-epileptic drugs for 7–10 days
- Preferred anti-epileptic drug is oral Levetiracetam
- Continuing prophylactic treatment longer than one week does not reduce late PTS/PTE

3. Post head-injury hypopituitarism (PHIH)

Pathophysiology

- Pituitary gland is connected to the hypothalamus via the pituitary stalk
- Blood vessels within the pituitary stalk are vulnerable to injury in TBI, leading to ischemia of the anterior pituitary lobe
- The posterior pituitary lobe is vulnerable to direct trauma that injures the axons projecting from the hypothalamus

Prevalence

- Highest in the acute phase after TBI, prevalence in acute phase is from 9–80%; long-term prevalence is ~30%
- Commonly affected hormones are: growth hormone deficiency, elevated prolactin, anti-diuretic hormone (ADH) deficiency leading to cranial diabetes insipidus, adrenocortiotropic hormone (ACTH) deficiency, and hypogonadism

Risk factors for developing PHIH

- Moderate or severe TBI, DAI, focal contusions
- Location of injury: basal skull, facial, sella turcica fractures
- Increased intracranial pressure

In acute post-TBI phase, it is of utmost important to identify **ACTH deficiency** (low cortisol, hypoglycaemia, hyponatraemia, hypotension) and **ADH deficiency** with cranial diabetes insipidus due to their high morbidity and mortality risks.

When to screen?

- At 3–6 months' post-TBI or if symptoms suggestive of hormonal imbalance-secondary amenorrhea, fatigue
- Basal blood tests for
  - Anterior pituitary function: 8 am cortisol, serum free T4, TSH, prolactin, FSH & LH, oestrogen (women) or morning testosterone (men). Insulin-like growth factor
  - Posterior pituitary: serum and urine sodium and osmolality
- Suggestive symptoms and equivocal screening blood abnormalities require referral to an endocrinologist for dynamic tests and further management

A clinical approach to TBI cognitive disorders

Impairments in cognition are found in virtually all survivors of traumatic brain injury (TBI) and are major causes of disability, reduced quality of life, and socio-economic burden. Commonly reported TBI-related cognitive impairments (CI) are diverse and have poor correlation with brain-imaged focal damage due to the diffuse nature of TBI, diaschisis, neurotransmitter downregulation, and secondary injury cascades. (Table 2)

Neuropsychological testing

Neuropsychological testing provides an appropriate assessment of cognitive deficits and can be regarded as an extension of neurological examination to more accurately evaluate higher brain functions. (Table 2)

Regarding neuropsychological testing for TBI patients:

- They should be performed when patients have emerged from PTA, and >6 months TBI having reached a plateau and can tolerate up to 120 minutes of testing with rest breaks
- They can give valuable information on relative strengths and weaknesses in an individual's cognition, and provide guidance for cognitive rehabilitation interventions
- They can be repeated to assess response to medication and remediation strategies or to assess the extent of recovery over time

Limitations of neuropsychological testing:

- Do not reflect the effects of compensatory memory strategies due to their specificity
- Do not equate to general measures of functional outcome
- Do not measure the impact of cognitive disability on daily functioning
- No one specific test or measure can accurately predict how well an individual with TBI will cope in everyday or vocational settings (Table 2)

Table 2. Common cognitive problems and tests used in clinical practice.

Domains	Clinical	Cognitive tests
Attention	• Arousal, task-specific attention • Divided attention • Attention span • Concentration	• WAIS-IV digit span subtest • Colour trails tests
Processing speed	• Reduced speed • Flexibility of thought processing	• WAIS-IV symbol search subtest • Trail making test A
Learning and memory		
Working memory	• Learning and remembering new information	• WAIS-IV digit span subtest
Verbal memory (immediate)	• Short-term memory	• RAVLT • WMS-IV logical memory I subtest
Verbal memory (delayed)	• Long-term memory	• RAVLT (delay trial) • RAVLT (recognition trial) • WMS-IV logical memory II subtest
Visual memory (immediate)	• Short-term memory	• WMS-IV visual reproduction I subtest
Visual memory (delayed)	• Long-term memory	• RCFT • WMS-IV visual reproduction II subtest
Language	• Problems finding words • Dysphasia • Impaired reading • Impaired writing	• Animal fluency • Naming task • COWAT

Visuospatial	• Vision • Diplopia • Visual fields • Visual inattention	• Clock-face drawing • Copying of simple figures
Visuo constructional	• Complex visual-spatial tasks • Copying block designs • Facial recognition tasks • Line cancellation tasks	• WAIS-IV block design subtest
Executive functioning		
Planning	• Planning and organization • Initiation • Follow-through • Monitoring outcomes	• D-KEFS tower test • BADS zoo map test
Reasoning	• Reasoning • Decision making	• WAIS-IV similarities subtest • WAIS-IV matrix reasoning subtest
Inhibition	• Inhibition	• D-KEFS colour-word interference test
Problem solving	• Unfamiliar problem solving • Dual tasking • Multi-tasking	• BADS key search test • Wisconsin card sorting test

Legend:
Wechsler Adult Intelligence Scale — Fourth Edition (WAIS-IV)
Wechsler Memory Scale — Fourth Edition (WMS-IV)
Rey Auditory Verbal Learning Test (RAVLT)
Rey Complex Figure Test
Behavioural Assessment of Dysexecutive Syndrome (BADS)
Delis-Kaplan Executive Functioning System (D-KEFS)
Controlled Oral Word Association Test (COWAT)

Cognitive rehabilitation after TBI

The role of cognitive rehabilitation is to improve and promote adaptive cognitive functioning in patients and enhance their participation in daily activities. The mainstay of cognitive rehabilitation involves non-pharmacological managements:

- Restorative — aims at restoring the impaired skills (e.g. remediation of memory deficits) and usually includes repeated practice of exercises of increasing difficulty

- Compensatory — aims at compensating for impaired functions through the usage of external aids (e.g. calendars, lists or memory notebooks and smartphones), environmental modifications (e.g. reduce distractors and use of visual cues) and behavioural strategies (e.g. use of feedback and reinforcements) (Table 3)

Table 3. Compensatory cognitive strategies for TBI.

Domains	Cognitive strategies
Attention	- Minimise potential distractions (e.g. background noises) - Encourage patients to focus on completing one task at a time - Avoid multi-tasking
Processing speed	- Pace themselves and allow more time to process, plan and organise their approach to tasks - Remind them to check over what they have done to increase accuracy
Learning and memory	- Repeat learnt information often to facilitate encoding and consolidation - Develop regular routines for tasks, which are repeated and rehearsed to encourage habit and automaticity - Use of external memory aids (phone calendar, reminders) to provide retrieval cues - Facilitate easier finding with fixed place for important personal effects (phone, keys, medications)
Language	- Use short and simple verbal or written instructions - Repeat instructions to facilitate understanding - Provide summary list of points to peruse at own time
Visuospatial	- Teach patients to follow a pattern of scanning to identify visual cues or landmarks when required, to navigate in less familiar environments
Executive functioning	- Encourage extra time to process, plan and break down tasks into smaller steps before deciding how best to proceed - Encourage patients to take time to reflect on their approach when stuck with problems - Provide guidance to consider alternative ways of doing things, as well as to seek feedback from external parties - Consider the best course of action in a systematic way - Avoid perseverating on an erroneous approach - In the case of impulsivity, learn behavioural strategies of delay (e.g. counting to 10) to slow down and allow more time to process or react to situations - Plan and organise approaches to tasks

Computer-aided cognitive rehabilitation (CACR) refers to cognitive training programmes delivered via computerised programs where targeted and repetitive training can be delivered to improve single or several different cognitive domains (e.g. attention, working memory). Progression in difficulty and duration are individualised.

Neuropharmacology in TBI rehabilitation

Medications used in acute to chronic TBI are often considered as "off-label" use, hence they should be used judiciously in conjunction with evidence-based approaches within a comprehensive goal-directed rehabilitation programme (Table 4).

- Prior to commencement of medication, reversible organic causes should be investigated for and treated (e.g. hydrocephalous, seizures, hyponatremia, metabolic derangements, sepsis, urinary or bowel retention, disordered sleep-wake cycles, fatigue, use of sedating medications)
- Rehabilitation team should jointly identify, target specific neurocognitive problems
- Serially monitor with standardised scales or patient/caregiver reported outcomes

Table 4. Common medication classes for cognitive disorders after TBI.

Problem	Medication	Dose (start/ max)	Common side effects	Comments
Hypoarousal	*Amantadine	100 mg BD/ 200 mg BD	Postural hypotension, dizziness, insomnia, nausea, GI intolerance	Epileptogenic: EEG recommended prior to starting
	*Bromocriptine	2.5 mg BD/ 10 mg BD	Postural hypotension, nausea, GI intolerance	
	LevoDopa/carbidopa	50 mg/25 mg BD	Headache/nausea	
	Modafinil	100 mg BD/ 200 mg BD		

Attention & processing speed	*Methylphenidate	5 mg BD/ 30 mg BD (0.3–0.5 mg/kg)	Tachycardia, hypertension, tremor, nausea, vomiting, anorexia	May worsen anxiety, glaucoma, abuse potential, MAOI therapy
	Atomoxetine	18 mg OM/100 mg OM	Dry mouth, nausea, insomnia	Closed angle glaucoma
	*Dextroamphetamine	5 mg OM/60 mg OM	Headache, irritability, insomnia, anorexia	Abuse potential, MAOI therapy, glaucoma
Memory For chronic TBI verbal domains	Donepezil	5 mg OM/ 10 mg OM	Nausea, diarrhoea, headache, insomnia	Caution in acute phase and seizures
	Rivastigmine	1.5 mg BD/ 6 mg BD	Nausea, diarrhoea, vomiting, anorexia, dizziness	
	Memantine	5 mg OM 10 mg BD	Headache, diarrhoea, dizziness	Irritability
Sleep	Trazodone	25 mg ON/ 200 mgON	Sedation priapism (males)	Antihistamine effects in higher doses
	Fluvoxamine	25 mg ON/ 150 mg ON	GI intolerance	SIADH, hyponatremia
	Mirtazapine	7.5 mg ON/ 45 mg ON	Weight gain, suicidality, orthostatic hypotension, hepatic dysfunction	SIADH, hyponatremia
	Melatonin	2 mg ON/ unknown maximum	Sedation	Onset may be delayed, serve at dinner time
	Amitriptyline nortriptyline	10 mg ON/ 150mg ON	Anti-cholinergic side effects, confusion, orthostatic hypotension	
Lack of initiation	Drugs in * are also useful in same doses			

(B.D. doses are usually given at 8 am and 12 noon or before 3 pm to avoid insomnia)

Disorders of consciousness and TBI

About 10% of brain injury survivors may enter a state of altered consciousness, termed "disorders of consciousness" (DOC) for periods exceeding 28 days.

These include:

- *Coma* [unwakefulness, eyes closed, reflex behaviours only]
- *Unresponsive wakefulness syndrome*, (UWS) or "vegetative state" (VS) [wakeful unawareness, reflexive behaviours only]
- *Minimally conscious states* (MCS) where clinical presentation includes clinical signs of consciousness, inconsistent ability to obey 1 step commands

Table 5. Distinguishing features of disorders of consciousness.

Disorder	Arousal/attention	Cognition	Command following	Motor function
Coma	No sleep wake cycles	None	None	None
Vegetative state	Present sleep wake cycles, intermittent wakefulness	None	None	Primitive reflexes or involuntary movements
Minimally conscious state	Intermittent periods of wakefulness	Inconsistent signs of behavioural awareness of self and environment	Inconsistent ability to follow 1-step commands	Localisation to noxious stimuli, object manipulation
Post-traumatic confusional state	Extended periods of wakefulness	Confused and disorientated	Consistent ability to follow 1-step commands	Full awareness, demonstrates use of common objects

- Differential diagnosis of DOC: locked in syndrome and akinetic mutism
- Emergence from MCS is signalled by recovery of functional communication, object identification, or object use
- Beyond these recovery stages, confusion, impaired attention, moderate to severe motor and functional disability usually persist

Diagnosis of DOC

- The mainstay of diagnosis is by clinical examination, with high misdiagnosis rates of about 40%
- Standardised scales used serially, such as the bedside JFK Coma Recovery Scale-revised (CRS-R) are useful to accurately quantify DOC and reduce misdiagnosis

Management of DOC

- DOC patients who have attained medical stability should be referred to multidisciplinary rehabilitation teams with specialized training to optimise diagnostic evaluation, prognostication, and subsequent management, including effective medical monitoring and rehabilitative care
- <u>Standardised neurobehavioral assessment</u> measures should be used serially (e.g. CRS-R)
- Where available, neurophysiological tools (quantitative EEG), functional imaging (functional MRI, tractal imaging, FDG-PET) should be integrated for multimodal evaluation to classify the states of consciousness
- <u>Therapeutic goals:</u>
    - Prevention and treatment of complications (e.g. infections, decubiti, paroxysmal sympathetic hyperactivity, spasticity, dystonia)
    - Neuro rehabilitation
    - Education support of the family
    - Long-term follow up
- <u>Pharmacologic management:</u>
    - Oral Amantadine given within 4–16 weeks of DOC onset in divided doses of 200 mg–400 mg daily for 4 weeks can safely and significantly hasten functional recovery from DOC
- <u>Non-pharmacologic management:</u>
    - 24-hour postural management protocols
    - Verticalization using tilt tables or stepping verticalization protocols supervised by physiotherapists
    - Management of spasticity and contractures

- Sensory stimulation programmes:
  - These involve multi-sensory stimuli (auditory, music, visual, tactile, olfactory, and gustatory) used serially at regular intervals
  - Insufficient to restore consciousness although CRS-R scores trended higher compared to usual care
- Neuromodulation and neurosurgical procedures:

  These are mainly research-based and include:
  - Transcranial direct current stimulation (TDCS) (non-invasive)
  - Repetitive transcranial magnetic stimulation (TMS) over the primary motor cortex (M1) or dorsolateral prefrontal cortex (non-invasive)
  - Deep brain stimulation (DBS) of the thalamic reticular nuclei (invasive)
  - Low intensity focused ultrasound pulse therapy (invasive)
  - Invasive vagal nerve stimulation (VNS) or transcutaneous auricular VNS (non-invasive)
  - Spinal cord stimulation (invasive)

Prognosis in DOC

- At 1 year post-injury, 52–75% may regain awareness
- At 1 year, 7–10% DOC patients may attain good recovery (GOS V)
- At 1 year, 45% have moderate to severe physical and cognitive disability

4

Spinal Cord Injury Rehabilitation

LUI Wen Li, CHAN Wai Lim William

Introduction to spinal cord injuries

How common is spinal cord injury (SCI)?

The incidence of spinal cord injury (SCI) is ~54 cases per million population in the United States (US) or about 17,810 new SCI cases.

Causes of spinal cord injury (SCI)

- Traumatic
  - Road traffic accidents
  - Falls
  - Assault
- Non-traumatic
  - Cervical spondylotic myelopathy
  - Prolapsed intervertebral disc
  - Spinal tumours (metastases to the spine is more common than primary spinal tumours)
  - Spinal cord infarction
  - Spinal cord vascular malformation
  - Spine infections (epidural abscess, spondylodiscitis)
  - Transverse myelitis

SCI clinical syndromes

i. <u>Central cord syndrome</u>: hyperextension injury from fall; background spondylosis; upper limbs more affected than lower limbs

ii. <u>Brown Sequard syndrome</u>: ipsilateral motor and proprioception loss; contralateral loss of pain and temperature

iii. <u>Anterior cord syndrome</u>: anterior spinal artery injury; flaccid paralysis; prognosis is poorer if there is spinothalamic function impairment–loss of motor and pinprick

iv. <u>Posterior cord syndrome</u>: dorsal column injury; loss of proprioception and vibration

v. <u>Cauda equina syndrome</u>: flaccid paralysis and sensory impairment of the lower limbs depending on nerve roots involved +/– areflexic bowel and bladder. Sacral reflexes, i.e. bulbocavernosus and anal wink will be absent

vi. <u>Conus medullaris</u>: terminal segment of the adult spinal cord; **mixed** picture of reflexic (due to conus injury) and areflexic signs (due to nerve root injury)

Rehabilitation assessment of SCI

History

- Demographics
- Comorbidities: past medical/surgical history
- Premorbid functional levels: Basic and Instrumental Activities of Daily Living (BADL), use of mobility or sensory aids
- Premorbid cognition and communication

- History of presenting illness
- Injury details where applicable:
  - Mechanism of injury (e.g. fall- level ground vs height, road traffic accident, industrial accident, assault, penetrating injury)
  - Type of injury
  - Associated injuries (e.g. polytrauma)
- Surgical intervention where applicable:
  - Complications of injury and treatment
- Specific conditions such as cardiovascular, musculoskeletal, rheumatological, pulmonary, and neurological conditions which may impact rehabilitation goals/exercise prescription
- Medication history
- Social history: genogram, family and friends support system, domestic helper, recreational activities and hobbies, spirituality, litigation, insurance, and compensation issues

- Home environment: living circumstances, identify environmental barriers, discharge placement, usual modes of transport
- Occupation history and requirements (e.g. driving, physical aspects)
- Family history

Current review of systems

- o In particular, enquire on symptoms associated with secondary impairments as a result of immobilisation, de-conditioning, weakness, sensory loss, autonomic dysfunction and pain, cognition, and mood

Physical examination

- o **International Standards for Neurological Classification of SCI (ISNCSCI)** (refer to next section)
- o Cardiovascular examination
- o Respiratory examination
- o Abdominal examination

- Review management thus far — including non-pharmacological and pharmacological management (e.g. analgesia, deep vein thrombosis (DVT) prophylaxis, sedatives, laxatives)
- Goal setting, estimated length of stay (ELOS)
- Discharge planning

International Standards for Neurological Classification of SCI (ISNCSCI)

- References for the 2019 revision of the International Standards for Neurological Classification of Spinal Cord Injury:
    - o ASIA and ISCoS International Standards Committee. The 2019 revision of the International Standards for Neurological Classification of Spinal Cord Injury (ISNCSCI)–What's new?. Spinal Cord 57, 815–817 (2019) https://lms4.learnshare.com/images/brand/204/Motor%20Exam%20Guide%20FINAL%20Feb%202020.pdf
    - o https://lms4.learnshare.com/images/brand/204/Key%20Sensory%20Points.pdf

- **Neurological level of injury (NLI)** — most rostral of the normal sensory and right and left motor levels
  - Motor level — the most caudal key muscle with a grade of 3 and above, provided the key muscles above it are graded 5
  - Lowest normal level for all modalities taken as sensory level on that side
- **Asia Impairment Scale (AIS): A to E**
  - Complete: (AIS A) absent sensory or motor function in the most sacral segment (S4/5) including absent voluntary anal sphincter and anal sensation
  - Incomplete (AIS B, C D, E): preserved light touch, pinprick, deep anal sensation at S4-5 or voluntary anal contraction present
  - (Worksheet: https://lms4.learnshare.com/images/brand/204/ASIA-ISCOS-Worksheet_10.2019_PRINT-Page-1-2.pdf
  - *Online algorithm: http://www.isncscialgorithm.com*

Common cardiovascular complications

(i) Autonomic dysreflexia (AD)

Andrew is a 41-year-old gentleman with chronic C7 AIS A spinal cord injury. Hs is currently being treated for urinary tract infection. He complains of headache, sweating and is very distressed. His face is flushed, and his blood pressure is 160/100, heart rate 60/min.

This case illustrates SCI-related autonomic dysreflexia. How can this be managed?

- Autonomic dysreflexia is a medical emergency for SCI patients
  - If left untreated, the rise in BP can result in cerebral haemorrhage, myocardial infarction, cardiac arrhythmias and seizures
  - Prompt recognition and urgent management are essential
- Pathophysiology
  - Results from massive sympathetic discharge in lesions at **T6 and above;** usually seen in complete injuries
  - Noxious stimulus below level of injury stimulates sympathetic system → splanchnic vasoconstriction → rise in BP; carotid baroreceptors cause reflex bradycardia, vasodilation above the level of lesion

- Signs and symptoms
  - Sudden rise in blood pressure > 20 mmHg above baseline with noxious stimulus
  - Headache
  - Tachycardia/bradycardia
  - Perspiration, flushing, piloerection above the level of injury
  - Blurred vision, pupillary constriction
  - Nasal congestion
- Management
  - **Aim to reduce BP, identify and remove the cause**
  - Sit patient upright, elevate head
  - Loosen all tight fitting clothing and devices
  - Flush indwelling catheter (IDC) if blocked
  - Change IDC–need to use local anaesthetic, (e.g. lignocaine gel) when inserting IDC
  - Monitor BP and pulse every 2–5 minutes during episode
  - Look for inciting stimuli and treat accordingly
    - Bladder: retention of urine, blocked catheter, urinary tract infection; urinary calculi
    - Abdominal causes: constipation, faecal impaction, appendicitis, cholecystitis, gastric ulcers
    - Skin issues: pressure ulcers, ingrown toenails,
    - Other causes: tight constricting clothing, limb fractures
    - Females: menstrual cramps, during labour/delivery
  - If BP does not decrease despite physical measures, administer medications: sublingual nifedipine 5 mg or sublingual captopril 25 mg; monitor BP until it returns to patient's usual baseline (this can be SBP < 100 mmHG in tetraplegics)

(ii) Venous thrombo-prophylaxis in SCI patients

Charles was involved in a road traffic accident 4 weeks ago and sustained a T6 AIS A spinal cord injury. He has been on subcutaneous Clexane injection since. He wonders if he needs to be on life-long Clexane.

- In individuals with SCI, venous thromboembolism has a high incidence and is potentially life-threatening
- Most of the new episodes of venous thromboembolism occur in the first two weeks after injury, with a significant decrease after eight weeks after injury
- Pathophysiology
    - Venostasis (failure of venous muscle pump)
    - Transient hypercoagulable state
    - Endothelial injury due to concomitant injuries
- Management
    - There is no role for routine screening for DVT
    - Mechanical prophylaxis: intermittent pneumatic compression devices with or without anti-thromboembolic stockings
    - Anticoagulation after assessing for any contraindications (i.e. bleeding risk)
        - Duration of anticoagulant thromboprophylaxis is variable:
            - **At least 8 weeks** in SCI patients with limited mobility and continued up to discharge from inpatient rehabilitation
            - Persons with chronic SCI who are hospitalised for medical illnesses or surgical procedures should receive thromboprophylaxis during the period of increased risk

Respiratory complications

Denise is a 50-year-old lady who was involved in a road traffic accident 3 months ago. She sustained a C5 AIS A spinal cord injury and required mechanical ventilation via a tracheostomy but has since been weaned off the ventilator and decannulated.

How does a spinal cord injury affect the respiratory system?

Introduction

- Respiratory complications after SCI are the leading cause of death
- Determinants of respiratory complications
    - Level of SCI, ASIA Impairment Scale (AIS)
    - Associated injuries (e.g. chest trauma)

- Other factors
  - Prolonged bed rest
  - Pain
  - Abdominal distension due to paralytic ileus

Aims of respiratory management

- Prevent complications
- Restore pulmonary function to the highest possible level by
  - Maximising breathing capacity
  - Enhancing cough ability

Anatomy and pathophysiology

- Respiratory muscles
  - Inspiratory muscles: diaphragm, external intercostals, accessory muscles
  - Expiratory muscles: abdominal muscles, internal intercostals
  - Innervation: diaphragm: phrenic nerve (C3, 4, 5)
- Respiratory complications after SCI
  - Respiratory muscle weakness, paradoxical breathing
    - Tetraplegics and high paraplegics: erect posture — diaphragm biomechanically disadvantaged
      - Nurse in supine position or use abdominal binder when upright
    - Decreased vital capacity
      - Vital capacity decreased to 20–60% predicted value in tetraplegics
  - Secretion encumbrance due to
    - Increased secretion production
    - Weak cough
      - Effective cough requires a large inspiratory volume and an expulsive expiration
      - Most complete tetraplegics require manually assisted cough due to weak intercostal and abdominal muscles

  - Bronchospasm
  - Pulmonary oedema
  - Pulmonary embolism
  - Sleep disordered breathing
  - Pneumonia, atelectasis and respiratory failure are more common in high tetraplegics

Assessment

- History and physical examination to assess for
  - Neurological level of injury/AIS
  - Respiratory symptoms
  - Underlying respiratory disorders
  - Oxygen saturation
  - Presence of paradoxical breathing
  - Cough strength (peak cough flow)
  - Lung volume (FVC/FEV1)
  - Symptoms of sleep disordered breathing: STOPBANG score/ Epworth Sleepiness Scale
- Review
  - Current method of respiratory management
  - Secretion load and character
  - Pneumonia/atelectasis episodes
- Investigations
  - Lung function test — forced vital capacity (FVC)
  - Peak cough flow (PCF)

Management

- Maximise breathing capacity
  - Abdominal binder when upright
    - Stabilises lower rib cage and improve diaphragmatic efficiency
  - Inspiratory muscle training (IMT) — devices that increase the resistive or threshold inspiratory load for improving strength

- o Glossopharyngeal breathing (GPB) — muscles of the mouth and pharynx used to propel small volumes of air through larynx; glottis is used to trap air into lungs to augment vital capacity
- o Lung volume recruitment (LVR): after breathing in maximally, augmented breath increases lung volume over and above vital capacity with use of breath stacking with bag valve mask

- Secretion management and enhancing cough abilities
  - o Measure PCF
    - PCF < 270 L/min is associated with poor cough and high risk of respiratory infection; requires manual cough assist and also LVR (via breath stacking with bag valve mask)
    - PCF < 160 L/min — despite LVR and manual cough assist — additionally requires mechanical cough assist with mechanical insufflation-exsufflation (MIE)
  - o Manual cough assist — increases peak expiratory flow rate (PEFR) during cough — assists cough by timing with patient's expiration
    - Contraindications — presence of inferior vena cava (IVC) filters, acute abdominal, or chest injuries
  - o MIE device (cough assist device) — provides deep inspiration (positive pressure) followed rapidly by controlled suction (negative pressure); rapid pressure change induces a high expiratory flow similar to a cough
    - Less traumatic than suctioning
    - Usually done 1–3 times daily

Neurogenic lower urinary tract dysfunction after spinal cord injury

Introduction

- Most individuals with SCI experience bladder dysfunction
  - o Even individuals who are ambulatory may have some form of neurogenic lower urinary tract dysfunction (NLUTD)

- Currently, renal failure is rare due to the improvement in management of NLUTD

- Pathophysiology
    - Disruption in the spinal cord between sacral nerves and the pontine micturition centre → inability to coordinate detrusor and sphincter for voiding and storage
    - Overactive bladder → overactive sacral reflexes +/– detrusor sphincter dyssynergia (DSD)
    - Underactive bladder → flaccid bladder, with loss of sacral reflexes
- Why is managing NLUTD important?
    - Symptoms can be distressing or embarrassing
        - Urinary incontinence
        - Urgency
        - Nocturia
        - Straining
        - Incomplete voiding
        - Urinary retention
    - Affects quality of life
    - Complications of NLUTD
        - Urinary tract infection
        - Autonomic dysreflexia
        - Hypercalciuria, stones
        - Upper tract deterioration

Goals of bladder management

- Preservation of upper tract function
- Improvement of urinary continence
- Preventing and treating complications such as UTIs, stones, strictures, and autonomic dysreflexia
- Improve quality of life
- Using a technique which is compatible with person's lifestyle

Assessment of a patient with NLUTD

- History
  - Level of injury, complete/incomplete injury
  - Urological history, pre-injury pattern of voiding
  - Current method of bladder emptying, awareness of need to empty bladder, ability to voluntarily void, urinary incontinence
  - Current drugs with possible influence on the urinary tract (anti-muscarinics, anticholinergics, TCA, alpha-blockers, alpha agonist)
  - Social history
- Examination
  - Saddle sensation
  - Anal contraction
  - Prostate size
  - UV prolapse in females
  - Sitting tolerance
  - Trunk control
  - Equipment (commode/wheelchair)
  - UL function/need for assistive devices for self IMC
- Investigations
  - Bladder diary: intake of fluids, voiding frequency, voided volumes, nocturnal voiding, urgency, incontinence episodes, and residual urine
  - Baseline upper tract evaluation: ultrasound (US) kidneys and bladder
  - Post-void residual (PVR) should be done in patients who are able to void
  - Urodynamic study (see section below)

Felicia is a 36-year-old lady with T6 AIS A spinal cord injury. She has just been transferred to the rehabilitation ward. She has had several failed attempts to trial off her indwelling urinary catheter (IDC) as she developed residual urine of 500 ml. How would we proceed to wean her off the catheter?

- Keep IDC until medical complications resolved
- Plan to trial off catheter when medically stable, absence of urinary tract infection and no further need for IDC (e.g. sacral sore management for

patients with incontinence, bladder irrigation, urological conditions (false passage), need for strict I/O monitoring) and if urinary output is <2 L/day

- Trial off catheter and remove IDC — typically done early in the morning
  - Pot Q4H potting and check post void residual urine
    - If patient is unable to void, to do intermittent catheterisation 4 hourly initially and note incontinent episodes in between
    - Adjust IMC schedule IMCs to ensure IMC volumes <500 ml
    - Avoid fluids after dinner to reduce the need of IMC in the middle of the night
  - Strict I/O (measure volume voided/weigh diapers)
  - Document any urinary leakages or urgency. If patient develops urinary leakages
    - Review fluids
    - Rule out UTI
    - Plan for urodynamic study (UDS) if urinary leakages or spontaneous voiding is noted
  - Monitor for AD with bladder filling
    - Monitor BP and heart rate half hourly
    - Abandon UDS if patient develops autonomic dysreflexia

Urodynamic studies (UDS)

- To classify the neurogenic bladder dysfunction
  - Urinary incontinence/storage failure may result from detrusor overactivity, atonic detrusor with overflow (high volumes), and pelvic floor insufficiency
  - Urinary retention/voiding failure may result from underactive/hypocontractile detrusor, outlet obstruction (persistent sympathetic tone, DSD; urethral stricture, enlarged prostate)
- Predict which patients will develop complications and require early intervention
- Identify factors contributing to incontinence for management

Management of bladder storage failure

- Neurogenic overactive bladder/low compliance (with or without DSD)
- Normal PVR volume does not mean the presence of a safe bladder
- UDS: high pressure filling phase, low compliance, low bladder capacity
- Bladder pressure >40 mmHg — risk of hydronephrosis
- Management: conversion of high-pressure bladder into low-pressure reservoir despite the resulting residual urine
    - Medications
        - Anti-muscarinics — oxybutynin, tolterodine, solifenacin, darifenacin
        - Tricyclic antidepressants, quaternary ammonium compound (e.g. trospium chloride); side effects: dry mouth, blurred vision, constipation
        - Beta 3 adrenergic agonist — mirabegron; side effects: hypertension, nasopharyngitis, headache, arthralgia, diarrhoea, abdominal pain
    - Empty bladder via intermittent catheterisation by self/carer
    - Consider intravesical Botulinum toxin A injection if oral medication fails/excessive side effects from medications

Management of voiding failure

- Underactive detrusor
    - Trial of bethanechol 10 mg P.O TDS to facilitate detrusor contraction; outcome is better when the bladder is partially innervated
    - **Discourage Crede or Valsalva manoeuvre** for bladder emptying due to the risk of high intravesical pressures and vesicoureteral reflux
    - Empty bladder (see next section on bladder emptying options)
- Outlet obstruction
    - Medications
        - Alpha adrenergic antagonist (phenoxybenzamine, terazosin, tamsulosin)
        - Spasmolytic agents (baclofen, diazepam; botulinum toxin injection)

    - Sphincterotomy/prostatectomy for BPH; urethrotomy/stent for urethral stricture
  - Empty bladder (see next section on bladder emptying options)

Bladder emptying options

- Intermittent catheterisation
  - Gold standard for management in patients with detrusor underactivity/a-contractility and those with detrusor overactivity
  - Frequency: start q4h — adjust frequency/fluid intake; maintain volumes at 400 ml
  - Clean technique allowed at home — use of soap and tap water to clean hands, no-touch technique. Sterile technique — full aseptic precautions when in hospital
- IDC
  - If unable to perform intermittent catheterisation or has high urine output
  - Temporary management of vesicoureteral reflux/hydronephrosis
  - Complications
    - Stones, urethral erosions, epididymitis, recurrent UTI, bladder cancer
    - Anticholinergics shown to reduce upper tract complications in chronic IDC
    - Consider suprapubic catheterisation for individuals with urethral abnormalities, perineal skin breakdown, body image issues, recurrent prostatitis, urethritis, or epididymo-orchitis

Long-term SCI bladder management

- Patients with high pressure bladders — renal US yearly to exclude hydronephrosis
- Serum creatinine yearly
- Urodynamic study when there are changes in signs or symptoms, new complications (recurrent UTI/autonomic dysreflexia)
- Renal function or upper tract deterioration

Urinary tract infections

Ian is a 20-year-old gentleman with T6 AIS A spinal cord injury. He has recurrent UTI and is currently on regular intermittent catheterisation. He now complains of increased spasticity and lethargy and his urine is cloudy. He also has non-blanchable erythema over bilateral ischial tuberosities and increased constipation. He wonders if he is having another episode of UTI again.

- Introduction
    - UTI is a common complication in individuals with NLUTD
    - UTIs can lead to complications such as
        - Autonomic dysreflexia
        - Increased spasticity
        - Renal complications
        - Hospitalisations
    - Diagnosis of UTI is challenging
        - Leads to over diagnosis of UTI given that asymptomatic bacteriuria is common
        - Atypical signs and symptoms due to altered sensation after SCI
            - UTI may present as
                - Increased spasticity
                - Autonomic dysreflexia
                - Constitutional symptoms (e.g. fever, lethargy)
                - Worsening or new incontinence
                - Abdominal pain
                - Malodourous or cloudy urine
            - The above symptoms are not specific to UTI and may also be due to other causes (e.g. constipation, blocked catheter)
- In a patient who presents with signs and symptoms that may be related to UTI
    - Rule out other possible causes
    - Send urine specimen for UFEME and culture
    - Treat with antibiotics if suggestive of UTI
    - Look for and manage complications of UTI (e.g. spasticity/autonomic dysreflexia)

- Recurrent UTI common complication for individuals with
  - Review bladder management
  - Reassess catheterisation technique
  - Assess for stones

Neurogenic bowel dysfunction

Joyce is a 40-year-old lady with cauda equina syndrome after a fall from height. She is distressed by the multiple episodes of bowel incontinence. Joyce avoids going out of the house and has incontinence associated dermatitis as a result.

What type of NBD does she have? How can her bowel management be optimised?

Introduction

- Most individuals with SCI have NBD
  - Constipation
  - Faecal incontinence
- Why is NBD important?
  - Bowel incontinence can lead to
    - Social isolation
    - Interferes with life activities
    - Decreased quality of life
  - Complications
    - Faecal impaction and constipation may cause:
      - Haemorrhoids
      - Megacolon
      - Autonomic dysreflexia
      - Worsening of spasticity
    - Bowl incontinence can increase risk of skin breakdown

Pathophysiology

- Reflexic bowel
  - Injury above the conus medullaris
    - Voluntary (cortical) control of stool disrupted

    - Increased tone and contractility of the rectum → reflex defecation and incontinence
    - Diminished relaxation of anal sphincter → retention of stool
  - Present anocutaneous reflex and bulbocavernosus reflex
  - Individuals with reflexic bowel have intact defecation reflex hence may benefit from
    - Use of gastrocolic reflex
    - Mechanical rectal stimulation (digital rectal stimulation)
    - Chemical rectal stimulation
- Areflexic bowel
  - Injury below the conus medullaris (usually L1 and below)
  - Areflexic at S2-4 — intrinsic myenteric plexus activity still present
  - Absent anocutaneous reflex and bulbocavernosus reflex
  - Reduced tone and contractility of rectum and external anal sphincter — increased risk of faecal impaction and incontinence

Aims of bowel program

- Regular passage of stool on a daily or every other day basis
- Adequate amounts of stool (moderate to large) with every bowel movement
- Bowel evacuation at a consistent time of day (am or pm)
- Complete emptying of the rectal vault with every bowel care session
- Soft, formed, bulky stools
- Completion of bowel care ideally in less than 30 minutes, but no longer than 1 hour
- No incontinence/bowel accidents

Assessment of an individual with SCI and NBD

- History
  - Level of injury, complete/incomplete injury
  - Pre-injury pattern of elimination
  - Current bowel status/bowel care
  - Current diet/fluids/medications

- Physical examination
    - NLI/AIS
    - Anal tone at rest/bearing down
    - Presence of deep anal pressure and anal contraction
    - Anocutaneous reflex, bulbocutaneous reflex
    - Haemorrhoids
    - Rectal/uterovaginal prolapse
    - Evaluate physical function — helps determine positioning during bowel care tasks
        - Hand function and dexterity
        - Sitting tolerance/trunk control

Management — individualised bowel management programme

- Lifestyle modifications
    - Adequate fluid and fibre intake, physical exercise
- Review medications that can cause constipation
- Oral medications to optimise stool consistency and colon motility
    - Commonly use medications include
        - Osmotic — PEG, lactulose
        - Stimulant laxatives — senna, dulcolax
- <u>Reflexic bowel</u>
    - Daily/EOD bowel clearance
    - Bristol Stool Form Scale 4 (smooth, soft)
    - Utilise gastrocolic reflex — consume food/beverage 30 min prior to bowel care
    - Rectal stimulants 10–15 min prior to digital rectal stimulation
    - Digital rectal stimulation
        - Gentle insertion and rotation of gloved finger at anus to stimulate recto-colic reflex; repeat every 5–10 min until stool evacuation is complete
        - Monitor for AD
        - Use lignocaine as lubricant for those at risk of AD
    - Manual evacuation of stool

- Areflexic bowel
  - Bowel clearance once or more times each day
  - Bristol Stool Form Scale score of 3 (firm)
  - Manual evacuation of stool

Pressure injuries

Ken is a 30-year-old gentleman with C7 AIS B SCI. He is currently being treated for a UTI which has resulted in increased urinary leakages and spasticity. He also has a stage 2 pressure injury.

What are factors contributing to his new pressure injury? How can further pressure injuries be prevented?

Introduction

- SCI patients are at high risk for pressure ulcers due to:
  - Impaired mobility
  - Impaired sensation
  - Prolonged sitting on wheelchair/lying in bed
  - Skin changes after SCI
- Pressure injuries are a serious preventable problem that affect health and function

Assessment of an individual with SCI who is at risk of pressure injuries/has pressure injuries

- History and physical examination to assess the risk factors for development of pressure injuries

Prevention of pressure injuries

- Institute pressure relief measures for all complete SCI
  - Begins in **acute phase** of SCI
- Perform daily visual skin inspection especially at areas prone to the development of pressure injuries (ischial tuberosities, sacrum, greater trochanters, malleoli, medial aspect of knees, occiput, calcaneum)

- Turning and repositioning
  - Institute 2 hourly turning
  - Avoid:
    - Overstretching and folding of skin/soft tissues
    - Shearing when individuals are repositioned or transferred
    - Positioning individuals who are side-lying in bed directly on greater trochanters
    - Donut-type devices
- Support surfaces
  - Pressure relief mattresses
  - Individually prescribed seating system designed to redistribute pressure
- Frequent and regular pressure relief in wheelchair
  - Side leans/forward leans
  - Tilt-in-space wheelchair
- Optimise nutritional status — meet individual needs for calories, protein, micronutrients, and fluids
- Patient education
  - Causes of pressure injuries
  - Prevention of pressure injuries
  - Daily visual skin inspection
  - Management of bladder/bowel incontinence
  - Turning and repositioning — frequency and duration
  - Pressure relief: frequency, duration, methods
  - Nutrition
  - Use and maintenance of support surfaces
  - When to inform the healthcare team

Management of pressure injuries

- Create a physiologic wound environment
  - Debridement of devitalised tissue
  - Wound care dressing

- Review condition leading to poorly-healing wounds
  - Bladder/bowel incontinence
  - Infection
  - Inadequate nutrition
  - Individuals with SCI and severe pressure injuries require about 5 kcal/kg of body weight per day more calories than those without pressure injuries
  - It is recommended for individuals with SCI and pressure injuries to have increased protein intake: 1.25 to 2 grams protein/kg
  - Support surface
  - Turning/repositioning
  - Transfer technique
- Refer individuals with stage III/IV pressure injuries for operative intervention
- Review pressure redistribution and support surfaces
  - Bed positioning
  - Bed support surfaces
  - Wheelchair and seating system
  - Pressure relief techniques

SCI and pain

Lina is a 30-year-old gentleman with C4 AIS A SCI. She complains of bilateral shoulder pain which is worse when side-lying and movement of her shoulders.

What is the approach to shoulder pain in a patient with high tetraplegia?

- Nociceptive pain
  - Musculoskeletal pain (e.g. glenohumeral arthritis, lateral epicondylitis)
  - Visceral pain (e.g. myocardial infarction, abdominal pain)
  - Other nociceptive pain (e.g. headache, surgical skin incision)
- Neuropathic pain
  - At level SCI pain (e.g. spinal cord compression, nerve root compression, cauda equina compression)

    - Below level SCI pain (e.g. spinal cord ischemia, spinal cord compression)
    - Other neuropathic pain (e.g. carpal tunnel syndrome, trigeminal neuralgia)
- Shoulder pain in tetraplegics
    - Neurological weakness and poor posture → muscle imbalance → anterior tightening; relative weakness of posterior stabilising muscles
    - Chronic impingement, rotator cuff pathology
    - Spasticity
    - Management
        - Proper positioning; wheelchair back support to improve posture
        - Avoid direct pressure on the shoulder when lying
        - Provide support to the upper limb at all times
            - Position upper limb in abduction and external rotation on a regular basis when supine
            - Avoid pulling on the arm when positioning individuals

Prognosis of spinal cord injury

Nova is a 26-year-old lady who was involved in a road traffic accident 3 months ago. She sustained a C6 AIS C spinal cord injury. She wonders if she will be able to ambulate in future.

What is the prognosis for spinal cord injury?

- Generally, most recovery occurs within the first 2 months post-injury, slower rate at 3–6 months, even up to 2 years post-injury
- Conversion of AIS at 12 months
    - Initial AIS A: 70% remained at AIS A, 17%, 6% and 7% improved to AIS B, C and D respectively
    - Initial AIS B: 23% remained at AIS B, 35% and 33% improved to AIS C and D respectively
    - Initial AIS C: 11% remained at AIS C, and 85% improved to AIS D
- Ambulation potential at 1 year post-injury can be predicted by
    - ASIA Impairment Scale (AIS) assessed within 72 hours post-injury
        - AIS A: 80–90% will remain complete; only 3% recover functional strength in the lower extremities

- AIS B: overall ambulation ranges from 10–33%
- AIS C: about 75% will become community ambulators; age and the amount of preserved spinal cord function below the lesion influence recovery of ambulation
- AIS D: majority will be ambulators

Appendix I. Functional outcomes by neurological level of injury

Domain	C1-C4	C5	C6	C7	C8-T1
Feeding	Dependent	Independent with adaptive equipment after set up	Independent, may need adaptive equipment	Independent	Independent
Grooming	Dependent	Minimal assistance needed with equipment after set up	Some assistance needed to independent with adaptive equipment	Independent with adaptive equipment	Independent
Upper body dressing	Dependent	Assisted	Independent	Independent	Independent
Lower body dressing	Dependent	Dependent	Assisted	Some assistance needed to independent with adaptive equipment	Independent
Showering	Dependent	Dependent	Independent to some assistance needed with equipment	Some assistance needed to independent with equipment	Independent
Bed mobility	Dependent	Assisted	Assisted	Independent to some assistance needed	Independent

Weight shift	Dependent in manual WC				
Independent with power	Assisted unless in power WC	Independent	Independent	Independent	
Transfers	Dependent	Maximum assistance	Some assistance to independent on level surface	Independent with or without board for level surfaces	Independent
Wheelchair propulsion	Dependent in manual wheelchair; independent with power wheelchair	Independent to some assist in manual WC, with adaptation on level surface; independent with power wheelchair	Independent with manual wheelchair with coated rims on level surface	Independent — except over curbs and uneven terrain	Independent

Appendix II

	T2-T9	T10-L2	L3-S5
ADL	Independent	Independent	Independent
Bowel and bladder care	Independent	Independent	Independent
Transfers	Independent	Independent	Independent

(See section on assistive technology for assistive devices used by individuals with SCI to enhance function)

5

Rehabilitation of the Geriatric Patient

THAM Shuen-Loong, PALANIAPPAN K

Introduction

Population aging, a global phenomenon, has been intensifying in recent decades as a result of declining birth rates and increasing life expectancy. Virtually every country is experiencing a growth in the number of older persons. This demographic shift has profound impact on healthcare, including rehabilitation needs. This is especially pertinent in Singapore, where we have one of the fastest growing aging populations in the world. Differential healthcare needs and issues exist amongst subgroups of older persons. For those 65 and older, the old-old (75–85 years old) and oldest-old (> 85 years old) groups are increasing in relative proportions and consumption of health services. High rates of frailty and disabilities are seen in these groups.

Disability and aging

Old age disability is observed as difficulties in performing of basic activities of daily living (ADLs) (such as feeding, bathing, toileting, dressing, grooming, transferring, and ambulating), or instrumental activities of daily living (e.g. telephony, shopping, meal preparation, housekeeping, taking public transport, managing medication and finances). A high rate of disability seen in the older persons results from the accumulation of health risks across a lifespan (e.g. diseases, injuries, chronic illnesses, exposure to environmental risks, social factors). Certain conditions are also found more frequently in the elderly (e.g. cancers, cardiovascular diseases). The gradual decline in physiological reserves (frailty) that accompany aging makes the body less able to withstand environmental or health perturbations, leading to disabilities.

As life expectancy improves, persons with disabilities (PWDs) are also more likely to develop premature age-related secondary conditions (directly or indirectly). For example, persons with cerebral palsy experience some premature physical aging 2 decades earlier than their healthy peers (e.g. pain, muscle stiffness, falls) due to abnormal or excessive strains with usual ADLs.

Defining geriatric rehabilitation

Geriatric rehabilitation aims to restore function or strengthen the residual functional capability, through diagnostic and therapeutic interventions, in aged persons who have disabling impairments. These are primarily focused on **function and well-being** (and not exclusively on disease), thereby preserving **functional independence**, and improving the **quality of life** in the elderly.

Conceptually, the principles of geriatric rehabilitation are similar to that of general rehabilitation. However, the recipients of the geriatric rehabilitation process show age-related characteristics (e.g. multimorbidity, multi-system frailties) and have needs that will require further thoughtful considerations (e.g. therapy techniques and intensity). The traditional definition of geriatric rehabilitation, which involved older persons with disabilities related to specific health conditions (e.g. stroke, arthritis), is now recognised as a part of a broader health strategy to improve functioning in the elderly.

Depending on rehabilitation needs, geriatric rehabilitation can be carried out in a variety of settings (e.g. acute hospitals, intermediate care facilities, rehabilitation units and community based settings). The beneficiaries of geriatric rehabilitation will typically have had prior acute or subacute decline in function. The ability to benefit from rehabilitation primarily depends on the extent of pre-existing disability (premorbid condition) and the severity of the presenting disability.

Chronological age per se should not be used to determine participation or ability to benefit from rehabilitation. Taking into consideration the above mentioned factors, individualised goals are set, and fulfilled through the efforts of a team of professionals working in an interdisciplinary fashion.

Physiological changes in aging

Physiological changes take place with aging in all organ systems (Table 1). However, there is great variability in the rate of decline for different organ system functions. An awareness of age-related physiological changes and understanding of their disease-related mechanisms of functional deterioration will aid the formulation of effective rehabilitation approaches in response to various disabilities.

Table 1. Physiological changes of aging and potential challenges during rehabilitation.

System	Physiological changes	Challenges during rehabilitation
Visual	• Blurry vision • Poor contrast sensitivity • Slower dark adaptation	• Difficulty performing tasks that relies on vision (including ambulation) • Requires adequate lighting for task performance
Hearing	• Decline in hearing acuity • Hearing loss	• Communication difficulties
Vestibular	• Vestibular disequilibrium	• Balance difficulties (affects reaching tasks, ambulation)
Respiratory	• Decreased lung elasticity (recoil) • Increased chest wall stiffness • Reduced respiratory muscle endurance • Less efficient gas exchange • Reduced lung volume and vital capacity • Less effective cough	• Increased work of breathing during effort • Easy fatigability and reduced ability to cope with effortful challenges
Cardiovascular	• Increased vascular stiffness => widened pulse pressure • Increased ventricular stiffness => decreased cardiac output • Degeneration of conduction system => heart beat irregularities • Valvular degeneration • Less efficient venous return • Decreased baroreceptor sensitivity • Decreased β-adrenergic responsiveness	• Exaggerated blood pressure response to effort • Poor heart rate response to effort (lowered maximum heart rate) • Easy fatigability • Orthostatic hypotension (arising from poor venous return and cardiac changes) cumbers vertical activities
Muscular	• Loss of muscle mass • Loss of muscle strength	• Inadequate muscular strength and endurance to perform physical therapy/exercises and tasks (e.g. ADLs)

Skeletal	• Decreased bone density • Degenerative joint changes	• Reduced joint flexibility hampers movement • Increased propensity for pain • Increased risk of fragility fracture
Neurological	• Cerebral atrophy • Altered cerebral autoregulation • Loss of speed of motor activities • Decreased sensation (including proprioception) • Cognitive decline (e.g. reduced short-term memory, information processing, memory retrieval)	• Balance difficulties & impaired coordination • Propensity for manifesting symptoms during postural hypotension • Requires more time to allow for information processing (e.g. giving instructions); requires a longer time for skill re-acquisition/task training
Urological	• Prostate enlargement in males • Less contractile bladder with hesitancy • Smaller less expansible bladder	• Nocturia can disturb sleep • Urinary frequency can interrupt rehabilitation training
Gastrointestinal	• Decline in taste and smell • Less healthy dentition • Small intestines absorb less of nutrients (e.g. vitamin B12, calcium, folic acid) • Colonic wall atrophy, slowed contraction, reduced mucin secretion	• Poor nutrition can adversely affect muscle health • Discomfort from chronic constipation affect performance in therapy
Sleep	• Fragmented sleep • Less deep sleep • Harder to fall asleep	• Propensity for poor sleep can affect performance (e.g. cognition), participation in therapy and mood

Rehabilitative management of the geriatric person

The delivery of rehabilitation to a geriatric patient will unlikely be solely focused on attenuating the disabilities stemming from frailty. The strategies employed may involve the following:

1. Rehabilitation for specific diseases (e.g. respiratory rehabilitation in chronic obstructive lung disease; stroke rehabilitation following cerebral infarction) (see respective relevant chapters)

2. Rehabilitation to mitigate/reverse the effects of bedrest and deconditioning (see chapter on "Deconditioning and Prolonged Immobilisation")

3. Rehabilitative management of frailty syndrome

The rehabilitative strategies for each of the above may not be unique to the domain and have considerable overlap. In the event of conflict, considerations to the condition of the patient, the context within which the patient is in, and patient's preference should be given. Prioritisation of interventions may need to be made in view of manpower, time, and cost constraints, as well as the patient's ability to cope. Owing to the general vulnerability of this population, geriatric rehabilitation often operates at close quarters with acute/subacute geriatric care (i.e. medical care).

Frailty syndrome

Frailty is characterised by aging-associated changes which, cumulatively and detrimentally, lead to decline in physiologic reserve and capacity across multiple body systems. As a result, the ability to cope with acute stressors and maintain physiological homeostasis is compromised (i.e. increased vulnerability). And this can lead to adverse health outcomes.

Clinical tools used to assess frailty include:

- The Fried Frailty Phenotype and Frailty Index — these are based on the phenotype and deficit accumulation models of frailty respectively, but utilisation of these tools can be time-consuming and laborious
- The Clinical Frailty Scale — a quick and simple judgement-based frailty evaluation tool used in the clinical setting
- Edmonton Frail Scale
- Hospital Frailty Risk Score
- The Comprehensive Geriatric Assessment (CGA) — possibly the best way to evaluate health and detect care needs in an elderly patient

Conceptually, frailty is distinct from disability and comorbidity (defined as additional diseases/conditions beyond the index disease). There exists a close relationship and considerable overlap amongst disability, frailty, and comorbidity with a synergistic impact of each on the other. Frailty and comorbidity each predicts disability, whilst disability exacerbates comorbidity and frailty.

Patients with a greater degree of frailty, even when functionally independent pre-morbidly, are susceptible to deconditioning during an acute illness (patient B compared to patient A in Figure 1). Rehabilitative interventions can help to reverse the level of dependency to independent levels of function (patient A). In situations where there is poor compliance, inadequate response to or an absence of rehabilitation, a new lowered baseline (patient B) can result. Potentially, this new reset baseline can fall below the threshold of independence, leading to a need for assisted care. (Figure 1)

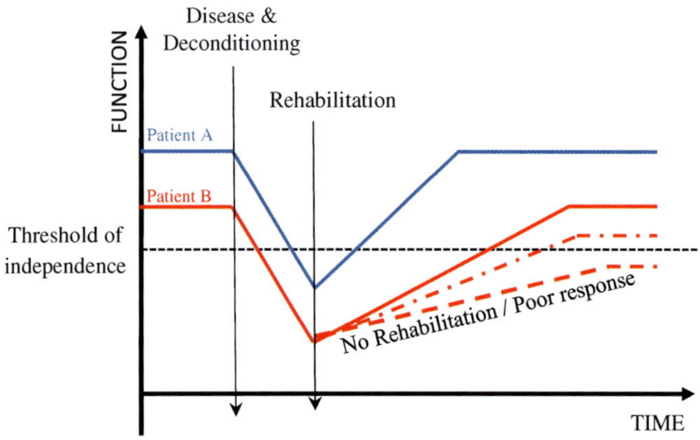

Figure 1. Functional outcomes following rehabilitation of the frail elderly.

Cognitive frailty

Cognitive frailty is a condition of diminished neuropsychological reserve where mild cognitive impairment and physical frailty co-exist. There is a close relationship between cognitive and motoric components of this condition. Evidence is emerging to reveal cross-talk between the brain and skeletal muscles, and their respective contributions to this condition. The brain is postulated to play a pivotal role in frailty syndrome. Reciprocally, physical activity has notable beneficial effects on the brain. One key significance of cognitive frailty is its reversibility (or potential for reversibility). Given its multi-factorial nature, multi-modal interventions (see below) are likely necessary for success.

Sarcopenia

Age-related sarcopenia is a syndrome of progressive generalised decline in muscle mass, strength, and quality, that leads to a deterioration in physical function and increased adverse outcomes (e.g. falls, dependency). The relationship between sarcopenia and frailty is complex and still incompletely understood. Sarcopenia has been considered a precursor syndrome, contributor, and even a physical manifestation of frailty syndrome.

Muscle mass and strength increase with growth in youth and young adulthood, being maintained in midlife and then decreasing with further ageing. In young adulthood (up to about 40 years of age), maximal levels are reached. Beyond the age of 50 years, loss of lean muscle mass (1–2% per year) and loss of muscle strength (1.5–5% per year) have been reported. Up to 50% of muscle mass can be lost by the 8th decade of life.

To date, there has been no universal consensus with respect to screening and diagnosis of sarcopenia. The European Working Group on Sarcopenia in Older People (EWGSOP), the International Working Group on Sarcopenia (IWGS) and Asian Working Group for Sarcopenia (AWGS) criteria aligned on the definition of sarcopenia: presence of low muscle mass, plus low muscle strength, and/or physical performance. EWGSOP2 criterion, a revision of the EWGSOP criterion, requires the detection of low muscle strength for probably sarcopenia, and a further evidence of low muscle quantity or quality for sarcopenia diagnosis. In the presence of diagnosed sarcopenia (i.e. low muscle strength and muscle quantity/quality), the finding of low physical performance is indicative of severe sarcopenia.

Exercise and nutrition remain the cornerstone of sarcopenia management (see below). Hormonal therapy (e.g. testosterone) is prohibitive due to its significant side effect profile, even though some evidence of its positive effects on muscle strength have been observed. Pharmacotherapy for sarcopenia reversal remains experimental at this juncture.

Managing frailty

a. Exercises/physical therapy

The management of frailty syndrome is challenging owing to its multi-faceted nature, as well as a paucity of evidenced interventions. Musculoskeletal decline (e.g. sarcopenia, osteoporosis) is a key feature of frailty syndrome. Exercise is integral to maintaining functional ability and attenuating several of the physiological changes (including musculoskeletal decline) that accompany aging. The adaptations to exercise and percentage improvement in physical fitness amongst the elderly are comparable to younger persons. But low aerobic capacity, muscle weakness and propensity for deconditioning, which are commoner in the elderly, can impact on their adoption or resumption of exercise.

Notably, physiologic aging does not occur uniformly in all elderly, that is, people with similar chronological age may differ in their responses to exercise. It is difficult to distinguish the effects of aging on normal function from the effects of deconditioning and/or disease. Functional assessments prior to exercise prescription can help to establish the baseline functional ability and monitor progress; (e.g. Senior Fitness Test, Short Physical Performance Battery, Usual Gait Speed, 6-minute walk Test and the Continuous Scale Physical Performance Test).

Evidence suggests that aerobic, resistance and/or balance training can improve physical function and attenuate the risk of age-related loss of physical function in the elderly. **Multicomponent** programs (incorporating elements of aerobic, resistance, balance, and flexibility exercises) were found to be more beneficial, especially when they can be integrated into the daily routine.

Various organisations, such as the World Health Organisation and American College of Sports Medicine, endorse **150 minutes** of moderate-intensity (or **75 minutes** of vigorous-intensity) aerobic activity and two or more days of strengthening exercises a week in the geriatric population. A sample of exercise prescription, as described in Table 2, may be appropriate for the elderly in good health, or at least with stable chronic disease conditions.

Table 2. Exercise recommendations for the elderly.

	Aerobic	Resistance	Flexibility	Balance
Frequency	3–7 days per week	2–3 days per week	≥ 2 days per week	1–7 days per week
Volume	20–60 minutes/ session (cumulative 150 minutes of moderate intensity or 75 minutes of vigorous intensity per week)	Begin with ≥ 1set of 10–15 repetitions; progress to 1–3 sets of 8–12 repetitions (for each of the 8–10 major muscle groups)	Hold stretch for 30–60 seconds per joint	1–2 sets of 4–10 different exercises that emphasise static and dynamic postures
Intensity	Moderate intensity (Borg CR10: 5–6) Vigorous intensity (Borg CR-10: 7–8)	Begin with light intensity (Borg CR10: ≤ 4) Progress to moderate (Borg CR10: 5–6) to vigorous intensity (Borg CR10: 7–8)	Stretch to the point of tightness or slight discomfort	Progressively increase level of difficulty: • Narrowing base of support • Perturbation of ground support • Reduce visual inputs • Reduce proprioceptive sensation • Moving the body's centre of mass from the vertical or stationary position • Adding a cognitive distractor or performing a secondary physical task whilst practicing balance

Exercise examples	Swimming, walking, stationary biking, aquatic exercise	Calisthenics, free weights, machines	Slow movements that terminate in static stretches for each muscle group; avoid rapid ballistic movements	Taichi, yoga, pilates

Borg CR10: Borg Category Ratio Scale

Beyond aerobic, strength, flexibility, and balance training, functional/task training (e.g. transfer training, participation in bathing and dressing) has a vital role in enhancing muscle health and function. Several programs, such as the Otago Exercise Program and Stay Active and Independent for Life (SAIL) program, incorporate several of the above-mentioned exercise elements and are evidenced to help mitigate falls in the elderly. Other falls programs, include additional components such as education and addressing fall hazards (e.g. home modification, prescribing adaptive equipment).

However, in the infirmed or severely deconditioned, even the minimal recommended amount of physical activity may be precluded or unachievable. Simple physical activities should still be encouraged and performed as much as tolerated and progressed with improved physical ability. In delivering exercise therapy for the elderly, and more so for the highly deconditioned and/or functionally limited, the following aspects should be given due considerations:

- Structured physical activities should be preceded by warm up exercises and end with cool down exercises (especially for patients with cardiovascular disease)
- Exercise intensity and duration should be initially light and gradually increased to target
- Exercise mode/type and progression should be individualised and tailored according to tolerance, limitation(s) imposed by the comorbid condition(s) and preference
- Exercise should be delivered and progressed according to overload principles and exercise training principles (e.g. in chair and bed rise tasks)
- Elderly individuals with significant cognitive impairment can still participate in physical activities but may require individualised assistance
- Progressive resistance/strength training, which is essential for sarcopenia management, should initially be supervised and monitored by personnel trained in exercise in the geriatric population and equipment used. Closed

kinetic chain, multi-jointed exercises are suitable for older adults starting resistance training

- Individuals with chronic conditions should be medically optimised, with an emphasis on exercises that are most beneficial to the limiting condition (e.g. aerobic training for persons with cardiovascular disease; weight-bearing and resistance exercises for persons with osteoporosis)

Physical and functional progress can be assessed as illustrated in Table 3.

Table 3. Common assessment tools for physical abilities.

Assessment tool	Assessed aspect
Modified Barthel Index	General function (activities of daily living)
Functional independence measure	General function (activities of daily living)
Timed up and go test	Functional mobility
30 second chair stand test/5 chair stand test	Lower limb strength and endurance
Dynamometer (grip)	Grip strength (reflection of upper body/overall body strength)
6 minute walk test	Aerobic capacity and endurance
10 metre walk test	Gait speed
Berg balance scale	Balance

b. Nutrition intervention

Aging is characterised by various modification of body composition (i.e. losses in muscle and bone mass, and accumulation of fat mass). Decreased total energy expenditure, increased insulin resistance, and increased muscle anabolic resistance to the anabolic effects of dietary amino acid substrates, have all been observed in the older adults. Aging and sedentary lifestyles have been linked with anabolic resistance, whereas exercise and higher dietary protein intake are beneficial to overcome this.

In the absence of any medical contraindication, a total daily protein intake of at least 1.0–1.2 g/kg body weight is recommended in healthy elderly aged 65 years and above. In active, exercising older adults, protein intake of more than 1.2 g/kg body weight/day is recommended. These need to be accompanied by replete energy intake (i.e. 30 kcal/kg body weight/day). Hospitalised elderly with acute or chronic disease will require a higher dietary protein intake of 1.2–1.5 g/kg body weight/day. In severe malnutrition, injury or illness, a daily intake of up to 2.0 g protein/kg body weight may be needed.

Nevertheless, nutrition intervention alone appears to have little effectiveness on sarcopenia reversal, unless combined with exercise intervention. Exercise (especially resistance training) is an effective stimulus for muscle protein synthesis.

Vitamin D is essential for maintaining muscle function and bone health. Daily oral intake of 800 IU is advised. Calcium intake should be increased in men older than 65 years and women older than 50 years of age. A daily intake of 1000–1500 mg of calcium is advised for bone health.

c. Multicomponent interventions

Apart from exercise and nutrition intervention, cognitive training interventions aiming to enhance attention, short-term memory, information-processing, problem-solving, perception organisation, and reasoning (e.g. puzzles, pen-to-paper tasks, video games) have been trialled with variable results. Care of other aspects contributing to frailty, are frequently embedded into many geriatric care programs as well (e.g. addressing polypharmacy, social isolation, smoking, alcohol abuse, oral health, chronic disease, and mood management).

Frailty is an ongoing affliction in the aged, and even with interventions of benefit, patient adherence is vital to ensure effectiveness. Applying principles of behaviour change to the frail elderly involves recognizing those components of frailty are treatable, understanding the intervention process and how it will improve outcome. To help the frail elderly make sustainable health behaviour changes, motivational strategies, while taking into consideration psychological, physiological, and economic barriers, will be necessary.

d. Geriatric care models/programs

When frailty, deconditioning and disease overlaps, it is almost impossible to discern the functional impact of one from the other. The hospitalised elderly frequently acquire functional impairments that require rehabilitation. In past decades, many geriatric rehabilitation systems/models were established to assist in the rehabilitative care of such elderly patients (e.g. the Acute Care of Elders (ACE–geriatric inpatient units) units, Geriatric Evaluation and Management (GEM — geriatric inpatient units) units, Hospital at Home (HAH) program, Hospital Elder Life Program (HELP)). Many variations of such models exist in different parts of the world. These programs differed largely in the components of care and site of care delivery. ACE units, more than others, had garnered some success in reducing functional decline and having patients discharge home.

Overall, the key attributes of a successful program should encompass the following elements:

1. Utilisation of Comprehensive Geriatric Assessment for evaluation of care needs
2. Multi-faceted care delivered by a multi-professional team
3. Inter-disciplinary care
4. Focus on rehabilitation and prevention of disability

At this time, strategies to prevent development of frailty are largely focused on addressing the drivers of functional declines: lack of regular exercise, malnutrition, cognitive impairment and development of chronic diseases, etc. Community-based interventions remain the focal point for such programs.

Recommended reading

- Cameron ID, Kurrle S *et al.* Geriatric Rehabilitation. In: Frontera WR (ed.) *DeLisa's Physical Medicine and Rehabilitation: Principles and Practice, 6th edition.* Philadelphia: Lippincott Williams & Wilkins (2020), Chap. 47, pp. 1054–1088.
- Izquierdo M, Merchant RA *et al.* International exercise recommendations in older adults (ICFSR): Expert Consensus Guidelines. *J Nutr Health Aging.* 2021;25(7):824–853.
- Liguori G *et al. ACSM's Guidelines for Exercise Testing and Prescription 11th edition.* Philadelphia: Wolters Kluwer (2022).

6

Cancer Rehabilitation

WONG Chin Jung, TAY Rong Jie Matthew, TEO Wee Shen

Introduction

With advances in cancer therapeutics, survival rates of patients have steadily increased. In many cases, cancer has been transformed from an acute illness to a complex and chronic disorder. However, survival does not always result in a disease-free state. Cancer and its treatment can cause physical and functional problems, as well as psychological sequelae, most of which may not be addressed adequately.

Cancer rehabilitation plays an important role in the care continuum of cancer survivorship. Dietz[1] first described a rehabilitation framework for cancer survivors at different stages of their illness. While this was described in the 1980s, it remains relevant and continues to guide rehabilitation strategies today:

1. Preventative rehabilitation: interventions that will reduce the effect of expected disabilities
2. Restorative rehabilitation: interventions that attempt to return patients to previous levels of physical, psychological, social, and vocational function
3. Supportive rehabilitation: interventions that help patients adapt to their disabilities and minimise debilitating changes from ongoing disease
4. Palliative rehabilitation: interventions that minimise or eliminate complications and provide comfort and support

Some common difficulties faced by the cancer survivors are illustrated in this chapter.

Case scenario

A 45-year-old lady was diagnosed with right breast cancer (Stage IIIA) 6 months ago and had a complete mastectomy and axillary clearance. She completed 33 sessions of adjuvant radiotherapy. She also completed a course of chemotherapy (doxorubicin and cyclophosphamide followed by paclitaxel) 3 months ago.

She was previously working in a customer service role, but has since gone on long-term hospital leave, initially due to cancer and later due to generalised weakness and fatigue. She does not use her right arm much due to some arm swelling and shoulder pain (secondary to increased weight of the arm).

She only does simple household chores whenever she is able to do so. She is unable to cook as she experiences numbness of her fingers and has hurt herself when chopping food. She also tripped and fell 1 month ago in the toilet when walking over a curb.

Cancer-related fatigue (CRF)

- Cancer-related fatigue has been defined by the National Comprehensive Cancer Network (NCCN) as "a distressing, persistent, subjective sense of physical, emotional, and/or cognitive tiredness or exhaustion related to cancer or cancer treatment that is not proportional to recent activity and interferes with usual functioning"
- Importantly, it is not proportional to exertion and may not be relieved by rest
- It is thought to be the most common symptom experienced in patients with cancer, ranging from 70% to 100%
- Though the etiology is still poorly understood, it may involve physiological and biochemical systems which may vary according to the type of tumour, stage of disease, and treatment
- It is also associated with pain, anaemia, medication side effects, emotional distress, sleep disturbance, nutritional deficits, and decreased functional status
- Persistent cancer related fatigue can affect quality of life, as patients are too tired to perform roles and activities

Screening

- Various assessment tools are available for screening, although most fatigue measures are self-reported and may not have the precision of objectives measures
- There are numerous measures available, including the brief fatigue inventory (BFI), sections of the EORTC Core Quality of Life questionnaire (EORTC QLQ-C30), visual analogue fatigue scale, medical outcome study short

form-36 (SF-36) and Functional Assessment of Chronic Illness Therapy-Fatigue (FACIT-F)

- *Cancer-related fatigue: ESMO Clinical Practice Guidelines for diagnosis and treatment* recommends that all cancer patients should be routinely screened for the presence and severity of fatigue from the point of diagnosis onward, at regular intervals during therapy and aftercare, and if clinically indicated

Evaluation

- A focused history and physical examination should be conducted if the fatigue is severe or has a negative impact on the patient
- Reversible medical conditions should be identified and treated. These include pain, anaemia, hyper/hypothyroidism, hypogonadism, deconditioning, steroid myopathy, adrenal insufficiency, infection, depression/anxiety, alcohol/substance abuse, insomnia, and cachexia
- Medications can contribute to cancer related fatigue (e.g. anticholinergics, antihistamines, anticonvulsants, neuroleptics, narcotics, antiemetics, beta blockers, antidepressants, muscle relaxants, and benzodiazepines)

Management

Address reversible causes:

- Pain and emotional distress should be detected and treated early
- If sleep disturbances are present, poor sleep hygiene behaviours should be identified and addressed
- A nutritional assessment is also useful in the presence of weight gain or loss. Fatigue symptoms may be improved with dietary modification to ensure adequate calorie intake, and correction of serum electrolytes imbalances
- Comorbiditics should also be reviewed, and optimally managed. For example, patients undergoing treatment for breast cancer are at risk of anthracycline-included cardiomyopathy. Minimising episodes of congestive failure can improve symptoms of dyspnea

Cancer-related fatigue

- Both the European society for Medical Oncology (ESMO) as well as National Comprehensive Cancer Network (NCCN) have recommended guidelines for management of CRF. Some of the common recommendations are summarised:

- o Patients should be educated about fatigue and its natural history. Most patients experience improving energy levels with time, especially if treatment is successfully concluded and medical related complications have resolved. Conversely, fatigue is expected to increase with disease progression
- o Energy conservation techniques should be taught to balance rest and activity during periods of high fatigue to maintain essential activities and goals. These include taking additional rest periods, pacing, prioritization, adopting proper postures during activities, delegation, and activity planning
- o Strong evidence exists for the role of exercise in reducing fatigue, which is the most effective treatment for cancer related fatigue. In general, patients should engage in exercise during or after cancer treatment, which can improve fatigue levels
- o There is growing evidence that physical exercise can attenuate systemic inflammation and improve CRF, allowing patients to become more capable of carrying out the activities of daily living
- o Exercise often consists of aerobic and/or resistance components in accordance with guidelines from the American College of Sports Medicine for cancer patients with the appropriate precautions
- o Nonpharmacological interventions include yoga, massage therapy, acupuncture, cognitive-behavioural interventions and bright white light therapy

Pharmacological agents

- There are limited studies on pharmacological agents for cancer-related fatigue and they remain investigational at current. There appears to be more support for these agents in more advanced stages of cancer
- These include psychostimulants like methylphenidate, corticosteroids, and modafinil. Even if these are used, clinicians should be still mindful to evaluate for specific morbidities that can contribute to fatigue

Re-evaluation

- There should be continued re-evaluation of the patient's fatigue during the course of the patient's disease and treatment

Peripheral neuropathy in cancer

- Apart from chemotherapy induced peripheral neuropathy, cancer can affect the peripheral nervous system, and can manifest as a radiculopathy, plexopathy, neuronopathy, mononeuropathy, polyneuropathy, neuromuscular junction disorder, myopathy, autonomic dysfunction, or a combination of these
- These can occur through various mechanisms, such as nerve compression, infiltration, hematogenous or lymphatic spread, meningeal or perineural dissemination
- Patients may already have an underlying neuropathy, or develop a neuropathy due to cancer, paraneoplastic syndromes, or treatment such as surgery, chemotherapy, radiation, immunotherapy, or stem cell transplants
- Electrodiagnostic studies can be useful for detecting subclinical neuropathic/myopathic processes, assessing for neuromuscular complications related to cancer, localizing the lesion(s), determining chronicity and severity, and understanding the pathophysiology and prognosis for neurological recovery
- Quantitative sensory studies, though not usually available, can provide information on small fibre involvement

Chemotherapy-induced peripheral neuropathy

- Chemotherapy associated peripheral neuropathy is the most common type of neuropathy in cancer patients
- Symptoms typically have a subacute onset, and occur in a distal, symmetric and length-dependent "glove- and stocking" distribution
- Sensory symptoms are more common than motor symptoms
- Side effects tend to be dose dependent, and can result in chemotherapy dose reductions and/or early discontinuation
- Symptoms may include pain, paresthesia, and dysesthesia
- Apart from a peripheral neuropathy, platinum-based drugs can damage the dorsal root ganglion, causing a pure sensory neuronopathy or ganglionopathy with a poorer prognosis. Platinum agents are commonly associated with a "coasting phenomenon" where symptoms can worsen for 2 to 6 months even after discontinuation of platinum-based drugs
- Taxanes and oxaliplatin can result in an acute neuropathy syndrome, in addition to chemotherapy induced peripheral neuropathy, which is largely reversible

- Vinca alkaloids often have some degree of motor involvement, in addition to sensory neuropathy

Table 1. Common chemotherapy drugs implicated.

Class of drugs	Examples
Platinum based drugs	Cisplatin, carboplatin, oxaliplatin
Taxanes	Paclitaxel, docetaxel, cabazitaxel
Other microtubule polymer stabilisers	Ixabepilone
Vinca alkaloids	Vincristine, vinblastine, vinorelbine, vindesine, etoposide
Other microtubule polymer destabilisers	Eribulin, brentuximab vedotin, ado-trastuzumab emtansine
Proteasome inhibitor	Bortezomib, carfilzomib, ixazomib
Anti-angiogenesis	Thalidomide, lenalidomide, pomalidomide
Others	Nelarabine, suramin, ifosfamide, pemetrexed

Evaluation

- Neurophysiological tests, as previously mentioned, can be used as objective quantitative assessment
- Clinical assessment requires patient history and risk factors such as relevant comorbidities, history of neuropathies, alcohol use, and toxin exposures
- The timeline of symptoms along with the chemotherapy regime, characteristics, and distribution should be elicited
- Physical examination should determine the clinical characteristics of the neuropathy (including sensory, motor, tendon reflex, autonomic assessment), functional impairment, and any related musculoskeletal findings
- There are also several proposed clinician-based grading systems, (e.g. NCI-Common Terminology Criteria for Adverse Events (CTCAE)), and patient-based grading systems, (e.g. FACT-Neurotoxicity Subscale (FACT-Ntx))

Management

- Serotonin-norepinephrine uptake inhibitors (e.g. duloxetine), tricyclic antidepressants (e.g. nortriptyline), antiepileptics (e.g. gabapentin), topicals (e.g. lidocaine patch), opioids

- To date, duloxetine appears to be the most promising in the setting of chemotherapy-induced peripheral neuropathy (CIPN). However, it is relatively contraindicated in patients on tamoxifen as it may inhibit conversion to its active metabolites via inhibition of cytochrome-P450 isoenzyme 2D6 (CYP2D6)
- Despite a lack of evidence, neurostimulation therapies and acupuncture have also been explored
- Management of functional deficits
    - Evaluation by a rehabilitation team
    - Adaptive strategies: orthotics, assistive/adaptive devices
    - Preventive strategies especially when lower extremities are involved (e.g. non-constrictive footwear, daily inspection of feet)
    - While there are no strong studies to support role of exercise in symptom mitigation with CIPN, exercise plays a role in addressing functional decline and deconditioning which are both common sequelae of CIPN

Cancer associated cognitive dysfunction in non-CNS cancers

- Cognitive dysfunction is a common complaint among cancer patients during or after chemotherapy
- Cognitive impairment can occur in both patients with brain tumours and in survivors without any brain involvement
- Cognitive dysfunction is widely reported to be associated with chemotherapy, but radiotherapy, hormonal therapy (e.g. tamoxifen, aromatase inhibitors, or androgens), and surgery can be associated with cognitive side effects
- The pathogenesis is largely unknown, though it is believed to be multifactorial, with direct and indirect effects on the central nervous system from the cancer and neurotoxic cancer treatment. Functional MRI studies have demonstrated changes in brain activity in cancer survivors with cognitive complaints
- Risk factors include previous cancer treatment, higher dose therapy or longer duration of therapy, concurrent chemoradiation, therapy delivered to the central nervous system, history of psychiatric illness, substance abuse, neurological disease or neurotrauma

- Common complaints are attention (e.g. focusing, concentration difficulties, distractibility, and difficulty multitasking), processing speed, executive function, learning and memory
- In chemotherapy induced cognitive dysfunction, studies suggest that short-term memory, working memory and verbal ability are most frequently affected, followed by visuospatial memory, executive functions, and attention span

Evaluation

- Reversible or confounding factors should be screened for, including emotional distress, sleep disturbance, fatigue, and pain
- Medications should be reviewed, as they may also contribute to cognitive impairment
- Imaging may be required for patients with new or focal neurological deficits
- There is no consensus on an effective brief screening tool or diagnostic criteria for cancer associated cognitive dysfunction, as current tools may lack adequate sensitivity
- Patient-reported measures of cognitive impairment is key in clinical assessment
- Hence, clinicians should attempt to elicit the characteristics and nature of cognitive dysfunction, along with the onset and evolution with time

Management

- Address reversible factors
- Review medications
- Compensatory strategies to minimise functional impact (e.g. reminders, calendars, smart phone alerts, keeping items in the same place)
- Cognitive retraining strategies
- Involvement of occupational and speech therapy to address specific functional limitations
- Cognitive behavioural therapy
- Encourage physical activity
- Relaxation, meditation, stress management, yoga

- Neuropsychological evaluation may be useful in select cases
- Studies on pharmacological treatment (e.g. methylphenidate, modafinil, gingko biloba, memantine, donepezil) are inconclusive at present
- Most patients with mild chemotherapy induced cognitive dysfunction will improve and return to their baseline within 1–2 years after cessation of treatment. However, cognitive dysfunction can persist long-term for a minority

Lymphedema in cancer

- Lymphedema may occur when lymphatic fluid builds up in soft tissue due to obstruction in the lymphatic system. Common causes include lymph node surgery, tumour invasion, tissue fibrosis (post-surgery or radiation-related)
- While many studies have been performed to elucidate potential risk factors to developing lymphedema, those with the strongest associations are increased BMI (especially > 25), more extensive lymph node surgery, more extensive surgical procedures, adjuvant treatment like radiation therapy (dose dependent) as well as sedentary lifestyle
- With chronicity, the protein rich lymph may lead to proliferation of fibrotic tissue and irreversible swelling of the affected region. Another complication that may lead to significant morbidity is cellulitis, as the trapped lymph fluid provides fertile ground for infections to occur
- It is important to understand that the risk of lymphedema does not diminish over time, but remains a lifelong risk. Hence the importance of early evaluation and management to minimise complications and morbidity
- From a rehabilitation perspective, lymphedema is associated with diminished function, diminished quality of life and management should be included in rehabilitation goal setting. Furthermore, management of the risk factors associated with lymphedema for (e.g. high BMI and sedentary lifestyle), are in line with rehabilitation principles

Evaluation

- The International Society of Lymphology (ISL) stages lymphedema from stage I–III, with the recognition of stage 0
- Stage 0: a subclinical condition where swelling is not yet evident despite the presence of impaired lymph circulation. Subclinical lymphedema may remain overt for months to years before clinical lymphedema develops

- Stage I: lymphedema involves early accumulation of protein rich fluid. Pitting may occur
- Stage II: involves more solid structural changes where limb elevation alone may not result in decrease in swelling anymore. Pitting may also gradually diminish
- Stage III: tends to be fairly disfiguring and is described as a state of lymphostatic elephantiasis. There may be trophic skin changes such as acanthosis, alterations in skin thickness, further deposition of fat and fibrosis with warty overgrowths developing
- Within each stage, a limited but nonetheless useful severity assessment has utilised simple excess volume differences assessed as minimal (> 5 to < 20% increase in limb volume), moderate (20–40% increase), or severe (> 40% increase)
- Factors like morbid obesity, lipodystrophy, venous congestion may complicate the clinical presentation. In the rehabilitation setting especially, in addition to diagnosis of lymphedema, there should also be care taken to exclude medical conditions like deep vein thrombosis, cellulitis, evaluate for concomitant musculoskeletal conditions that may affect ability to undergo further lymphedema care (e.g. frozen shoulder, axillary cording)
- If diagnosis is uncertain or greater prognostic/therapeutic certainty is required, usage of imaging or other forms of investigation may be helpful
  - Ultrasound studies to exclude deep vein thrombosis
  - Lymphoscintigraphy
  - Magnetic resonance imaging, computed tomography
  - Early detection of tissue changes (useful especially in stage 0) include usage of bioimpedance spectroscopy, bioimpedance analysis, tissue dielectric constant
  - Infrared perometry
  - Water displacement volumetry
- In the rehabilitation setting and depending on severity, lymphedema is usually also associated with functional impairments and other musculoskeletal conditions. In addition to determining presence of lymphedema and cellulitis during history and physical examination, attention to weight gain and exercise habits during history taking also aids in management. During physical examination, where applicable, the musculoskeletal condition proximal and distal to the region of lymphedema should be assessed

  - For example, breast cancer survivors with breast cancer surgery and axillary lymph node clearance with resultant lymphedema of the ipsilateral side, may also go on to develop shoulder pain related to adhesive capsulitis, rotator cuff impingement. If the surgery was fairly recent, there may be presence of axillary cording
- Finally, Health Related Quality of Life (HRQOL) and patient perceptions of self-efficacy assessed by validated disease specific instruments and visual analog scales of patients with lymphedema should be used together with physiological measures to evaluate the effects of treatment

Management

- The treatment of lymphedema can be divided into conservative and operative approaches
  - Conservative approach. The cornerstone of care continues to be complete decongestive therapy (CDT) comprising of manual lymphatic massage strategies, muscle pumping exercises, compression with bandages and subsequently compression garments. Other possible modalities of intervention include low level laser therapy, elevation of affected limb, kinesiotaping
  - The benefits of education, counselling, proper skin care are also not to be underestimated
  - In Singapore, patients are referred to trained allied health care professionals in both the private setting and public healthcare institutions for CDT and interventions listed above
  - Unfortunately, there are very few one stop programs for lymphedema care in Singapore. While competent allied health professionals are able to deliver CDT, the holistic care that is required in rehabilitation of lymphedema remains at the discretion of the primary physician. Lifestyle factors like exercise and diet, psychosocial well being, body image concerns, assessment for concomitant MSK conditions (e.g. adhesive capsulitis, axillary cording) that affect function, are often overlooked in a busy clinic setting
  - Pharmacological management. Diuretic agents are of limited use during the initial treatment phase of CDT and should be reserved for patients with specific comorbid conditions or complications
  - Operative approach. These are usually performed to improve lymph return. However, in advanced stages, they usually require

long-term combined physiotherapy and/or other compression after the procedure to maintain edema reduction. They tend to be adjunctive to CDT, or if CDT was unsuccessful

- o Lymphovenous anastomosis, liposuction and lymph node transfer operations with lymphedema therapy and compression are effective when used to treat appropriate lymphedema patients and performed by an experienced surgeon

Exercise and safety concerns in cancer rehabilitation

- Physical activity has been shown to have a multitude of health benefits including lesser side effects from cancer treatment, improved quality of life and even survival
- Physical Exercise Across the Cancer Experience (PEACE). The PEACE framework introduced by Courneya and Friedenreich summarises how physical exercise may impact the patient throughout their cancer journey. It describes how physical exercise may affect cancer outcomes throughout the phases of prevention, detection, buffering, coping, rehabilitation/palliation, health promotion, and survival
- As it is easy to implement and generally safe, more clinicians are recommending exercises to their patients
- Due to impairments arising from either cancer or cancer treatments, a very common concern is whether it is safe to undergo various forms of exercises. Concerns with how exercise may impact on immunity or worsen pain and fatigue are common
- On this note, there are several guidelines written that support the safe prescription of exercise in cancer patients/survivors (e.g. American College of Sports Medicine (ACSM), Exercise and Sports Science Australia)
- Despite the shifting paradigm towards exercise in cancer patients, there is still room for improvement when it comes to physical activity/exercise amongst cancer survivors in Singapore

Evaluation

- In general, there are very little contraindications to physical activity. Patients in intensive care for example could still benefit from simple exercises involving range of motion to the limbs to minimise joint contractures

- ACSM recommends that no prior assessments are required to start a light intensity walking, progressive strength training, or flexibility program in survivors with no significant co morbidities
- Despite this, some important factors should be considered as patients' conditions may change, or they might have different goals. For example:
  - Older survivors and/or survivors treated with chemotherapy induced peripheral neuropathy may benefit from a standard assessment of balance and mobility to assess fall risk
  - Patients with cognitive dysfunction may require constant supervision as they undergo exercises
  - Patients with chronic medical conditions, cardiovascular diseases may need further screening and even comprehensive physical examination prior to undertaking an exercise program
  - The National Comprehensive Cancer Network (NCCN) has recommended that patients with no significant comorbidities may safely undertake exercise programs according to their recommendations, without any prior screening or assessment
  - For patients with conditions like ongoing chemotherapy, joint arthritis, lymphedema, poor bone health for instance, evaluation by medically trained personnel is recommended
- Depending on comorbidities, basic history taking and physical examination may suffice. In more complex cases (e.g. cardiotoxicity following anthracyclines), further investigations or even cardiology review may be warranted

Management

- ACSM guidelines describing what exercise goals to achieve in cancer survivors are similar to those in the general population. The difficulty lies in the titration of exercises given concomitant conditions like fatigue, neuropathy, ongoing chemotherapy to name a few. In addition, specific precautions need to be observed in certain conditions (e.g. lymphedema, bone metastases). An example of general ACSM guideline recommendations is tabled below (Table 2):

Table 2. General ACSM guideline recommendations.

Exercise	Aerobic	Resistance	Flexibility
Frequency	3–5 days per week	2–3 days per week with at least 24 h rest interval	2–3 days per week, daily if possible
Intensity	Moderate to vigorous level, using HR_{max}, RPE or talk test to help monitor	Moderate (10 to 15 repetitions). Start with a weight you can lift 10 to 15 times but lift it only 3 to 5 times. Gradually build up to 10 to 15 repetitions	Move through range of motion (ROM) as tolerated
Time	≥ 150 $min{\cdot}wk^{-1}$ of moderate-intensity aerobic activity, 75 $min{\cdot}wk^{-1}$ of vigorous aerobic activity, or an equivalent combination of both for adults	At least 1 set of 8–12 reps. Increase up to 3 sets. Involve all major muscle groups	10–30 s hold for static stretching. Repeat up to 3–4 times
Type	Rhythmic, weight-bearing exercises using the large muscle groups, such as walking, swimming, and cycling	Use machine weights first. These help with balance problems. As strength and balance improve, add free weights or resistance bands. Your body can be used as resistance with push-ups and sit-ups	Stretching or ROM exercises for all muscle groups
Importance	Achieve 20–60 min of moderate-to vigorous intensity per session. It can be done all at once or be broken up into a few sessions of at least 10 minutes each	Necessary to improve or maintain muscle and bone, ability to function and promotes good health	Yoga, tai chi, and pilates help with balance, flexibility, and relaxation. These can be incorporated as part of flexibility, stretches. Yoga also helps reduce swelling and improve immune system function during breast cancer treatment

- Some common considerations for exercise in cancer patients (Table 3)

Table 3. Common considerations for exercise in cancer patients.

Considerations	Recommendations
Bone loss/bone metastases	Avoid movements that place an excessively high load on fragile skeletal sites. These include: high-impact loads, hyperflexion or hyperextension of the trunk, flexion or extension of the trunk with added resistance, and dynamic twisting motion • Preventing falls must also be a goal of therapy, since falls play an important role in fracture etiology • Be aware of signs and symptoms of bone metastases in survivors, as well as common locations where these occur (i.e. spinal vertebrae, ribs, humerus, femur, pelvis). Bone pain can be an initial sign of skeletal metastases thus, exercise trainers should refer survivors who report pain back to the medical team for clinical evaluation before continuing exercise
Lymphedema	• ACSM recommends use of compression sleeves for resistance training based on NCCN guidelines and Position Statement of the National Lymphedema Network • Being overweight or deconditioned have been associated with a higher risk of developing cancer-related lymphedema in observational studies
Ostomy	• Empty ostomy bag before starting exercise • Weight lifting/resistance exercises should start with low resistance and progress slowly under the guidance of trained exercise professionals. People with an ostomy may be at an increased risk of parastomal hernia. To regulate intra-abdominal pressure, correct lifting technique and good form is required. Avoid use of a Valsalva manoeuvre • Modify any core exercises which cause excessive intra-abdominal pressure, namely a feeling of pressure or observed bulging of the abdomen • Those with an ileostomy are at increased risk of dehydration. Ensure optimum hydration prior, during and after exercise • Those doing contact sports or where there is a risk of a blow to the ostomy may wish to wear an ostomy protector/shield
Peripheral neuropathy	• Stability, balance, and gait should be assessed before engaging in exercise; consider balance training as indicated • Consider alternative aerobic exercise (stationary biking, water exercise) rather than walking if neuropathy affects stability or use treadmill with safety handrails • Resistance training recommendations: o Monitor discomfort in hands when using hand-held weights o Consider using dumbbells with soft/rubber coating, and/or wear padded gloves o Consider resistance machines over free weights

Stem cell transplantation	• Home-based exercise encouraged if patient is neutropenic or prone to infections • A full recovery of the immune system recommended before return to gym facilities with the general public • Start with light intensity, short durations but high frequency and progress slowly • Exercise volume (intensity and duration) should be adapted on a daily basis based on the individual's presentation • Watch for skin graft vs host disease, which may lead to skin tightening, contractures. Flexibility exercises are encouraged • Watch for anaemia and low platelet counts and exercise due caution
Sun safety	• In addition to melanoma survivors, survivors of cancer at other primary sites may be at increased risk for secondary skin cancers if exposed to sun for prolonged periods during PA • Exercise professionals should recommend that cancer survivors engage in sun protective practices when exercising outdoors • Concerns with photosensitivity with patients on chemotherapy. Recommend indoors exercises for patients on chemotherapy • Concerns with photosensitivity with patients on radiotherapy/post radiotherapy. Recommend avoiding direct sun exposure for 4–6 weeks post radiation at least

- In summary, exercise is a key component in rehabilitation of many cancer-related impairments. It is safe to undergo if appropriate precautions and screening are undertaken.

  Goals of exercise have to be ascertained and regular reviews are recommended to ensure the exercise prescribed remains relevant and safe to undergo

References

1. Dietz JH. Adaptive rehabilitation in cancer: a program to improve quality of survival. *Postgrad Med.* 1980;68(1):145–153.

Recommended reading

- Denlinger CS, Sanft T *et al.* Survivorship, version 2.2018, NCCN clinical practice guidelines in oncology. *J Natl Compr Canc Netw.* 2018;16(10):1216–1247.

- Hayes SC, Newton RU *et al.* The exercise and sports science Australia position statement: exercise medicine in cancer management. *J Sci Med Sport.* 2019;22(11):1175–1199.
- O'Dell MW. In: Stubblefield MD (ed.) *Cancer rehabilitation: principles and practice 2nd edition.* (2018).

7

Rehabilitation of the Lower Limb Amputee

TJAN Soon Yin, ONG Poo Lee

A person with lower limb amputation faces many challenges. Besides losing a limb, he or she has to learn to overcome limitations in self-care, mobility, and societal participation (e.g. employment, sports and leisure). The care of an amputee requires close coordination between members of a multi-disciplinary team through different phases of the amputee's recovery. The overwhelming cause for lower limb amputation in Singapore is vascular complication secondary to diabetes mellitus (DM). Diabetic lower limb amputees are also at risk of further amputation. Hence, the goal of rehabilitation is both restorative and preventive.

The ICF (International Classification of Function) provides a good framework for assessing functional deficits of the lower limb amputee and should be used together with the biopsychosocial model for holistic assessment, goal setting, and management.

Phases of rehabilitation for major lower extremity amputation (LEA)

Table 1 shows the phases and timelines in the rehabilitation of DM patients with a below knee amputation (BKA), starting from the day of amputation. Patients with above knee amputations (AKA) usually need a longer period of rehabilitation.

These proposed timelines may be influenced by the following factors:

a. Physical condition prior to rehabilitation

b. Stability of medical condition(s)

c. Cognitive ability

d. Social support

e. Motivation

f. Logistic constraints

The clinical milestones define the goals to be achieved as the amputee progresses from one phase to another. Education and reconditioning are facets of rehabilitation care that run through all phases rehabilitation. These timelines can potentially be used as a systems-based outcome measure to compare amputee rehabilitation programs offered by different providers.

Table 1. Rehabilitation phases, milestones and timelines of DM patients with BKA.

	Pre-prosthetic			Prosthetic		
Phase	Pre-operation	Immediate post-operation	Pre-prosthetic, casting	Prosthetic gait training	Community integration	Maintenance
Timeline	Days before operation	3 weeks	4–6 weeks	8–12 weeks	Up to 6 months	3 years
Important clinical milestone	Start patient education, reconditioning	STO (removal of surgical stitches)	Stump shaping	Competent use of prosthesis consistent with prognosis and goal	Return to societal participation	Life span of prosthetic system, preparing for next prosthesis

Types and levels of lower limb amputation

The types and levels of lower limb amputation are shown in Figure 1.

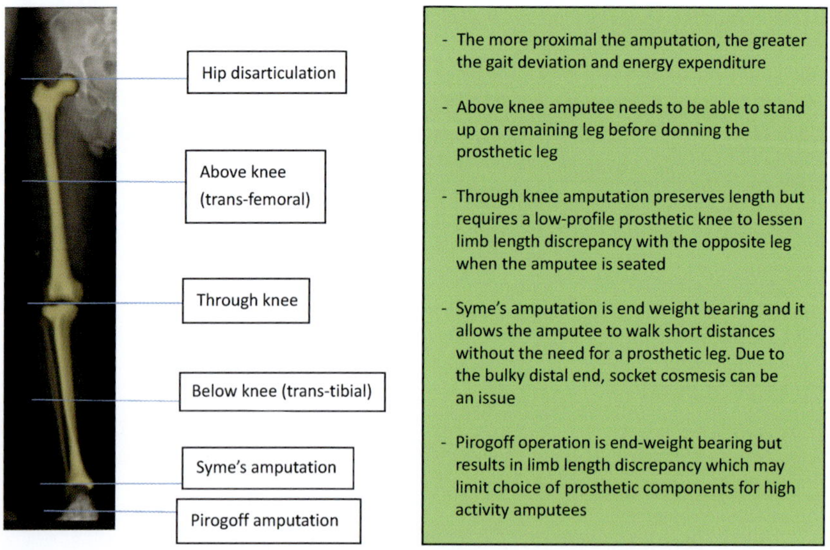

Figure 1. Common anatomical levels for LEA and prosthetic implications.

The Medicare Functional Levels (Figure 2), or simply and more commonly called K levels, is the most commonly used classification system for lower limb amputees according to walking ability. Patients with different K levels use prostheses with different components (as shown in Figures 3 and 4).

Medicare Functional Levels (MCFL)/K Levels & Goal-setting

- K0 – Non-Ambulator
- K1 – Homebound Ambulator
- K2 – Limited Community Ambulator
- K3 – Unlimited Community Ambulator
- K4 – Sports and Heavy Manuel Prosthetic User

The K classification is used ***after*** an amputation to stratify walking ability/goal. It determines the type of components chosen for the prosthesis (lower K users need stability whereas higher K users will benefit from components that enhance mobility). K3 is characterised by the ability to walk with variable cadence and negotiate environmental barriers. Return to work usually means achieving at least K3 in order to take public transport. K4 users may need to have more than one prosthesis to fit demands of different activities (running prosthesis is different from walking prosthesis).

Figure 2. MCFL K classification — the Central Functional Classification for LEA.

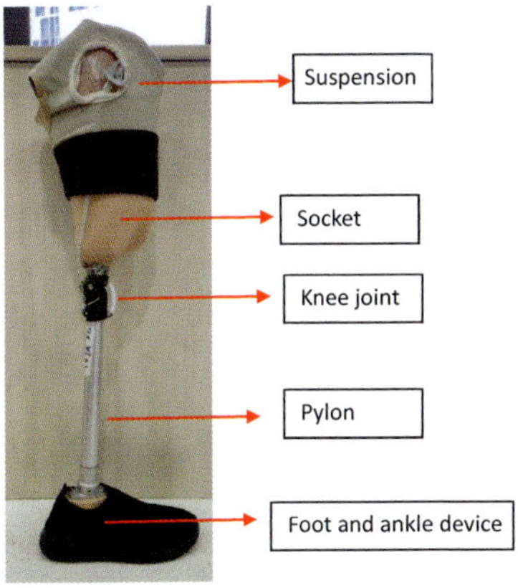

	K1	K2	K3
Common Component Choices	- SAKL (Semi-Automatic Knee Lock) - Safety Knee - SACH (solid ankle cushioned heel) foot	- 4 Bars Multiaxial Knee - Dynamic Response System (DRS ankle-foot)	- Pneumatic/ Hydraulic Knee with/without computer chip - DRS ankle-foot - Shock absorptive or adaptive ankle-foot
Notes on Usage	- Emphasises knee stability over mobility - Users walks with less or no knee flexion - Difficult to climb stairs	- Allows more mobility but needs user to have good proximal muscle control	- Allows easier cross terrain mobility - Usually used with Silicone Inner Knee sleeve suspension - Computer knee allows for climbing stairs foot over foot without need to hold rails

*K4 users need custom and separate prostheses for different functional demands

Figure 3. Prosthetic component choices and usage in AKA prosthesis.

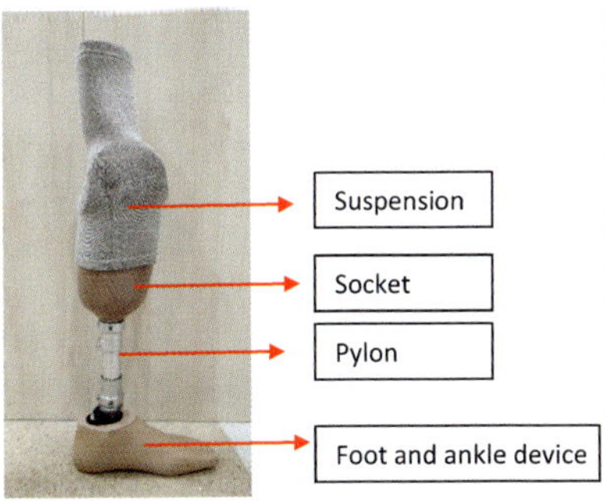

	K1	K2	K3
Common Component Choices	- Mulley strap - SACH (solid ankle cushioned heel) foot	- Silicone knee sleeve suspension - Dynamic Response system (DRS ankle-foot)	- Pin - lock suspension - Suction suspension - DRS ankle-foot - Shock absorptive or adaptive ankle-foot
Notes on Usage	- Emphasises on stability over mobility - Ease of donning especially for user with poor hand dexterity	- Allows more mobility with better suspension - Knee sleeve may cause skin allergy and heat for some user	- Allows easier cross terrain mobility - Needs good cognition and hand dexterity for donning and doffing of suspension

*K4 users need custom and separate prostheses for different functional demands

Figure 4. Prosthetic component choices and usage in BKA prosthesis.

Prognosticating ambulatory status after amputation

An amputee's premorbid ambulatory status is the most important factor in prognosticating ambulatory status after amputation. This can be classified using AMPSIMM (Amputee Single Item Mobility Measure). The AMPSIMM scores from 0 to 6 with higher scores indicating better mobility. A score of 6 indicates the ability to walk in the community without the need for ambulation aids at unlimited distance.

Amputee Single Item Mobility Measure (AMPSIMM)

AMPSIMM Level	Description
0	Bedridden mostly, house bound and require help for household transfer and mobility
1	Wheelchair user at home but not get out into community
2	Wheelchair user at home and community
3	Walking at home with aid, use wheelchair in community
4	Walking in community with ambulatory aid (e.g. cane, crutches, walker)
5	Walking in community without aid but limited distance (e.g. one block equivalent).
6	Walking in community without aid, unlimited distance

Source: Norvell, Czerniecki et al. (2016).

A person who has the ability to walk within 6 months prior to amputation i.e. AMPSIMM 3 and above, has a good prognosis to be a functional prosthesis user. Other factors include the patient's medical (cardiorespiratory, neuromuscular, cognitive, and special senses, especially vision), psychosocial and financial status.

It is essential for the healthcare team to be able to predict the patient's ability to walk with a prosthesis. Prescribing a prosthesis when it is not needed leads to unnecessary waste of financial resources. On the other hand, not prescribing a prosthesis when it is necessary may deny the patient a chance for prosthetic ambulation and better integration into society.

Table 2 shows the positive and negative predictors of ambulatory status after a LEA. Generally, a patient who is younger, has a distal level of amputation with trauma as the cause of the amputation tends to have a better outcome. The transtibial amputee, when compared to the transfemoral amputee, retains sufficient sensory and motor capacity due to preservation of the knee, and is able to maintain better dynamic stability during ambulation. Early referral to rehabilitation is also associated with better ambulatory outcome. Education plays an important role throughout the rehabilitation journey of the amputee. This include care of the preserved foot especially in diabetic patients, proper shoe wear, stump care, skin care, lifestyle management, and proper donning and doffing techniques.

Table 2. The positive and negative predictive factors for walking ability following lower limb amputation.

	(+) Predictive factors	(–) Predictive factors
Age	Age < 60	Age > 60
Level of amputation	Unilateral or transtibial	Bilateral or transfemoral
Cause of amputation	Traumatic	Vascular
Premorbid motor function	Independent in ambulation and self-care Ability to stand on one leg	Require assistance in basic care
Comorbidities	No significant comorbidities	End-stage renal failure, hemiparesis, cardiac failure, and respiratory disease
Others	Previously employed and has good social support	Cognitive or mood disturbances

It is important to recognize that prognostication for prosthesis use/prescription can change when the patient suffers further complications (e.g. a unilateral BKA patient may have the prognosis revised downwards if he/she suffers another amputation or another disease such as stroke).

Pre-prosthetic phases: pointers for functional restoration and preventive care

The pointers in Table 3 and 4 ***should be read with the clinical milestones stated in Table 1 in mind.*** Where necessary, clinical pointers introduced in earlier phases should continue into later phases.

Table 3. Clinical pointers from provider, patient, and system of care perspective in amputee rehabilitation.

	Pre-operation	Immediate post-operation	Pre-casting
Provider (health care team)	- Assess functional needs and refer to rehab team (e.g. physiotherapist) - Assess vascular reserve of unaffected leg KIV vascular scan	- Follow updated strict wound management protocol, use correct wound products - Properly assess and chart pain as fifth vital sign. Refer to acute pain team if necessary	- Make provision to use Removable Rigid Dressing (RRD) early by liaising with surgeon performing amputation - Make provision to use compressive stump socks (e.g. Juzo) when contraindications are absent

	- Assess risk of developing chronic pain; yellow flags like low mood, prior history of chronic pain, prolonged duration of pain and poor pain coping mechanisms are more important predictors of development of chronic pain than intensity of pain	- Assess nutritional status especially need for protein supplement	- Monitor and document stump circumference using standardised methods - Make provision on wheelchairs/orthosis to promote prevention of knee contracture for BKA
Patient	- Encourage to share worries and expectations - Educate on need to start reconditioning	- Participate in exercises including self-exercise taught by therapist - Learn desensitization for stump pain and phantom pain - Introduce Diabetic Foot Screening (DFS) for remaining leg	- Learn positioning techniques to minimise stump edema - Learn methods to prevent knee contracture for BKA
System	- Provision of e-learn/ patient education materials for amputee rehabilitation - Possible blanket referral to rehabilitation/Allied Health Professionals (AHP) team	- Provision of e-learn/ patient education materials for suitable bed exercises - Consider having doctors/ward nurses learn DFS and education	- Provision of standard protocol to activate Prosthetic service for casting of prosthesis - Provision of standard methods to assess and document ambulatory goal and prognosis for amputees

Table 4. Prosthetic phases: pointers for functional restoration and preventive care.

	Gait training	Community integration	Maintenance
Provider (health care team)	- Explain clearly gait training goals and plans to amputee/ caregiver	- Be familiar with various community resources available (e.g. financial support schemes, peer-support	- Consider serving as volunteers to promote activation for amputees

	- Follow clinical precautions and communicate challenges to rehabilitation team for trouble shooting - Provide gait training at correct intensity and specificity within limits of timeline and patient progress	resources, return to driving, return to work, adaptive sports vendors) - Work out SMART goals with clear outcome measures together with amputees and care givers	- Learn to provide correct information and resources to help amputees stay active in community
Patient	- Encourage to learn self-exercise at home/community - Practice DFS and good foot care especially with DM diagnosis	- Encourage to stay connected, voice challenges and explore services as activated patients - Learn good DM control and adopt good lifestyle choices	- Encourage to participate in planning finances for prosthesis remake - Encourage to participate actively in community including serving to help other new amputees
System	- Provide alternatives to outpatient clinic visits (e.g. home therapy) to ensure training compliance - Ensure team members use standardised training and documentation procedures to facilitate outcome tracking	- Encourage an ecosystem to support patients' integration and independence in community (e.g. wheelchair repair resources, peer support group, education forums, or online resources to allow amputees to stay connccted) - Provide ongoing onboarding/e-learning to ensure new healthcare practitioners are updated on work processes/resources	- Continue to explore provision of financial and other resources to support amputees' recovery journey in community - Analyse and act on identified gaps in service/education/advocacy for amputees' activation

Common problems faced by the LEA

Table 5 below shows common problems and their management during different phases of amputee rehabilitation. A proper assessment of the cause and type of pain should be performed prior to treatment. Stump pain (or residual limb pain), needs to be differentiated from phantom limb sensation and phantom limb pain.

Table 5. Differential diagnoses and management of common problems in LEA.

	Issues	Causes	Management
Pre-prosthetic	• Stump pain	• Could be generated from bone or soft tissue, infection, or neuromas	• Evaluate underlying cause of pain • Adequate post-op analgesia and education
	• Phantom pain	• Exact etiology is uncertain; irritation of severed nerve endings is one of the postulated causes • Usually occurs 2 to 3 months after amputation or even later	• Desensitization technique — massage/tapping/vibration • Use of stump shrinker • Mirror therapy, virtual reality therapy, mental imagery • Transcutaneous electrical nerve stimulation • NSAIDs, opioids • Anticonvulsant (e.g. gabapentin)
	• Wound breakdown	• Infection, trauma, blister formation, stump oedema	• Proper dressing and hygiene • Recheck vascular status if the patient is diabetic • Education on wound care • Monitor and control blood sugar (for diabetes patient) • Regular review by healthcare professionals
	• Emotional and psychological issues	• May occur at any phase of rehabilitation journey • Reaction varies greatly and depends on many factors • Loss of limb, function, self-image, relationship • Distorted body image	• Early referral to rehabilitation, including psychologist for supportive counselling, coping strategies, and maximising function • Cosmetic prosthesis to restore body image for those not suitable to use functional prosthesis

Prosthetic/ gait training	• Stump pain	• Skin-related issues (e.g. swelling, pressure ulcers, blister, and infection) • Extrinsic cause such as poor socket fitting may contribute to stump pain	• Good stump hygiene • Avoid wearing prosthesis once any skin issues are detected and treat appropriately • Ensure proper socket fitting and alignment of prosthesis • Maintain stable body weight
	• Gait deviation	• Prosthesis factor and/or user factor • Ill-fitted socket (too loose/too tight) • Unequal prosthesis length • Muscle weakness (e.g. hip abductor, hip extensor) • Underlying pathology, (e.g. osteoarthritis, stroke, etc.)	• Clinical gait analysis by experienced healthcare professional to identify the underlying cause • Adjustment of prosthesis, change of interface, or recast of socket may be necessary
Maintenance	• Prosthesis wear and tear	• The lifespan of each component varies and may range from 6 months to 3 years	• Regular review by prosthetist at least once every year for component check and safe use of prosthesis

The socket of the prosthesis is where the stump of the lower limb amputee sits in. A good fitting socket allows for even distribution of the amputee's body weight towards pressure tolerant areas and avoiding areas that can cause pain, skin, or bone damage (e.g. distal tibia in BKA amputee). It also allows the lower limb to be secured firmly. A poorly-fitted socket can lead to a variety of issues including pain, blister formation, skin breakdown, ulcer and increased risk of falls. One also needs to understand the proper use of socks and liners with the prosthesis. Socks can prevent friction between the skin and socket or interface. However, using many layers of socks to compensate for a loose socket increases the risk of skin breakdown due to shear forces between the stump, socks and the socket.

Community re-integration

Lower limb amputees face an uphill task returning to work. Just like all other disabilities, the longer a person is away from work, the lesser the success rate for returning to work. Thoughtful consideration and conversation about returning to work should commence early in their rehabilitation journey i.e. pre-prosthetic phase. Hospital and/or community-based services can further facilitate this endeavour, as would support groups (e.g. amputee support group).

Lower limb amputees who wish to return to driving would need to be re-assessed for fitness to return to driving. For more information, please refer to the chapter on "A Holistic Approach to Return to Work and Driving After a Disability".

Participation in sports and exercise is beneficial for promoting physical and mental health. The American College of Sports Medicine's recommendation of moderate intensity aerobic activity for a minimum of 150 minutes per week and resistance exercise (of the major muscle groups) twice or more a week also applies to amputees. A lower limb amputation does not limit an individual from taking up or continuing a sport. Adaptations may be required in selected sports (e.g. wheelchair tennis). Some sports, such as swimming (even though aquatic prosthesis may sometimes be used), may be enjoyed without additional equipment. The success of para-events, such as the Paralympics, is an indication of society's growing interest, support, and recognition of disabled individuals in sporting contexts.

Amputee clinic at foot care and limb centre

At Tan Tock Seng Hospital, the amputee clinic was set up as a multidisciplinary team clinic at Foot Care and Limb Design Centre. It is represented by the rehabilitation physician, prosthetist and orthotist, physiotherapist, podiatrist, occupational therapist, and medical social worker. It is a one-stop centre that allows the amputee rehabilitation team to review and manage the amputee patient within the same session without the need for multiple visits. Such a team-based service allows for better management and support of the amputee, be it medical, psychosocial, or financial.

Recommended reading

- Clinical guidelines for the pre and post operative physiotherapy management of adults with lower limb amputations — second edition. *British Association of Chartered Physiotherapists in limb Absence Rehabilitation*. 2017. Retrieved from https://www.bacpar.org/resources/healthcare-professionals-resources/pre-and-post-op-guidelines/
- Life after amputation: what to expect for the new amputee. *PAM Health*. Retrieved from https://pamhealth.com/company/company-updates/life-after-amputation-what-to-expect-for-the-new-amputee
- The orthotics & prosthetics virtual library. *Digital Resource Foundation for the Orthotics & Prosthetics Community*. Retrieved from https://www.oandplibrary.org/

8
Cardiopulmonary Rehabilitation

NG Valerie Zhi-Yan, HENG Cheryl, SWAPNA Tony

Introduction

Patients with cardiopulmonary issues may have problems with breathlessness, fatigue, and anxiety, leading to a reduced quality of life. They may also have questions or issues with their compliance to treatment plans. Cardiopulmonary rehabilitation is a holistic intervention that combines education and exercise to help these groups of patients cope with their symptoms and management of their disease.

The goals and benefits of exercise in cardiopulmonary rehabilitation are:

- Establish a patient-controlled and safe aerobic exercise program
- Reduce dyspnea, anxiety, and depression
- Maximise cardiovascular and pulmonary capacity and mechanical efficiency
- Provide guidelines for safe activities and work by energy conservation strategies
- Improve quality of life and activities of daily living (ADLs), mobility, and social activities
- Control risk factors for coronary artery disease (CAD)
- Decrease the frequency of hospitalisations

General components of cardiac and pulmonary rehabilitation

Cardiopulmonary rehabilitation is usually delivered by a multidisciplinary team of doctors, nurses, and allied healthcare professionals. (Figure 1)

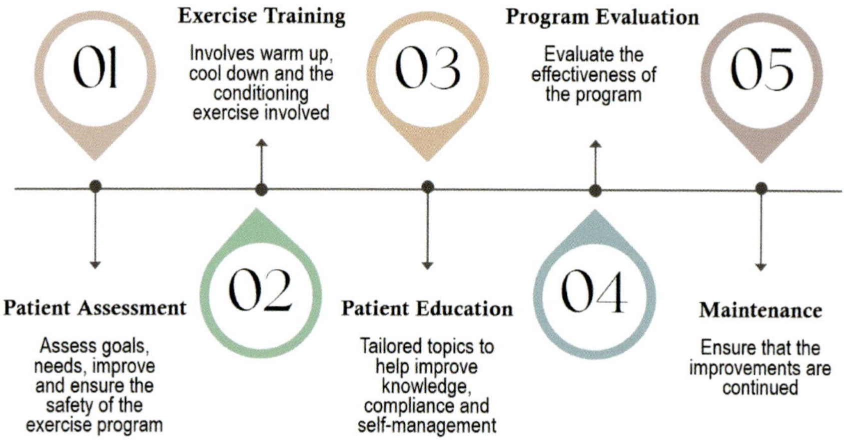

Figure 1. Components of a rehabilitation program.

1) Patient assessment

Baseline patient assessment helps to identify patient needs and goals, risk stratify the patient and ensure that exercise prescription and education are tailored to the individual. In some cases, it helps to evaluate if there is a potential need for supplemental oxygen. The 2 types of assessments are summarised in Table 1.

It is important to screen for **contraindications** to cardiopulmonary exercise in the following situations:

- Unstable angina, active pericarditis/myocarditis, recent acute myocardial infarction, symptomatic congestive heart failure
- Severe aortic stenosis, severe pulmonary hypertension, untreated pulmonary embolism

Table 1. Baseline patient assessment.

Medical assessment	Fitness assessment
• Risk factors, symptoms or signs of active cardiac or pulmonary disease • Premorbid and current activities and endurance levels • Cognitive and behavioural status, mood, vision, nutritional status • Physical impairments that may affect exercise training Laboratory data, electrocardiogram (ECG) or echocardiographic abnormalities to institute special precautions as needed • Optimization of pharmacologic management	• Endurance, strength or balance assessments (e.g. 6 minute walk test, 5 times sit to stand test, 10-meter walk test, etc.)

- Uncontrolled diabetes mellitus
- Acute systemic illness or fever
- Resting heart rate > 120/bpm (tachycardia)
- Uncontrolled resting blood pressures: SBP > 200 mmHg and DBP > 100 mmHg
- Orthostatic BP drop of SBP > 20 mmHg during exercise
- Uncontrolled atrial or ventricular dysrhythmia, 3rd degree atrioventricular (AV) heart block
- New onset of resting ST displacement > 3 mm
- Neurologic (severe cognitive impairment, evolving neurological deficits) or orthopaedic (e.g. acute arthritis, active pain, or fractures) problems which may be worsened by exercise

2) Exercise training

Exercise training involves warm up, cool down, and the conditioning exercise itself (could be endurance, strengthening or both).

The **FITT** principle is used for exercise prescription: **Frequency, Intensity, Time, and Type**.

The **Karvonen formula** calculation is used to determine the **Target Heart Rate** training zone.

The Karvonen formula is your heart rate reserve (HRR) multiplied by the percentage of intensity plus your resting heart rate. e.g. **Target Heart Rate Training Zone = Resting HR + (% Intensity × [maximum HR – resting HR])**.

For example, a 50-year-old with a resting heart rate (RHR) of 60 at 50% intensity would calculate as follows:

- Maximal HR = 220 – 50 (age in years) = 170
- HR reserve (HRR) = 170 – 60 = 110 × 50% = 55
- Target Heart Rate (THR) = HRR + resting HR = 55 + 60 = 115

For patients on beta blockers, Karvonen formula may be less suitable and arbitrary estimated THR as +25 beats above RHR can be used depending on patient's cardiac status (e.g. THR = 60 (RHR) + 25 = 85).

The difference in exercise prescription and monitoring between cardiac & pulmonary patients for are listed in Table 2 below.

Table 2. Exercise prescription and monitoring.

	Cardiac rehabilitation	Pulmonary rehabilitation	General fitness
Frequency	• Aerobic exercise 3–5 times a week • Strength training at least 2–3 non-consecutive days a week	• Endurance training 3–5 times a week • Strength training at least 2 days a week performed on non-consecutive days	Aerobic exercise: • 3–5 times a week for improving cardio-respiratory fitness • 5–7 times a week for weight loss and maintenance of weight loss • Strength training: 2 times a week for each major muscle group
Intensity (aerobic exercise/ endurance training)	• 40–60% of heart rate reserve • 3–4 on Modified BORG Dyspnea* Scale	• 3–4 on Modified BORG Dyspnea* Scale	• Moderate intensity (40–59% HRR) and progress to vigorous (> 60% HRR) • 3–4 on Modified BORG Dyspnea* Scale *(refer to Table 3 below)*
Intensity (strength training)	60–70% of 1 repetition maximum, performed for 8–12 repetitions (if prescribed by a qualified trainer)		
Time	• Aerobic exercise: 30 minutes • Strength training: 1–3 sets; 8–10 different exercises focused on major muscle groups	• Endurance training: 30 minutes. If patient is deconditioned, can break up into sets of 10 minutes with short rests if required • Strength training: 2–4 sets, 8–12 repetitions	Aerobic exercise: • 30–60 minutes for general exercise (accumulating to at least 150 minutes a week) • 60 minutes for each session for weight loss and maintenance of weight loss Strength training: 8–12 repetitions
Type	**Aerobic/endurance:** walking, cycling, swimming, machines (e.g. treadmill, cross-trainer, etc.) **Strength training:** upper limb and lower limb strengthening exercises using body weight, additional weights, machines and/or resistance bands. (there needs to be at least **3–4 exercises** per session involving major muscle groups in the upper and lower body as well as the core)		
Monitoring	• Heart rate • Breathlessness	• Breathlessness • Sp02 Levels (keep > 88%)**	• Heart rate • Breathlessness

**Refer to Table 3 below for the Modified BORG Dyspnea Scale*

***Unless advised by physician*

To monitor exercise intensity, either the Modified Borg Dyspnea Scale or the talk test can be used.

For the Modified Borg Dyspnea scale, patients are asked to rate their current level of difficulty of breathing on a scale of 0–10, where 0 is causing no difficulty and 10 is maximal difficulty. For the talk test, during a moderate-intensity activity, patients should be able to talk but not sing.

Table 3. Modified BORG Dyspnea Scale.

Rating	Modified Borg Dyspnea Scale
0	Nothing at all
0.5	Very, very slight (just noticeable)
1	Very slight
2	Slight
3	Moderate
4	Somewhat severe
5	Severe
6	
7	Very severe
8	
9	Very, very severe
10	Maximal

Performing a warm up and cool down before and after exercise is highly recommended. Doing a warm up helps to prepare the body for exercise and reduce the risk of injury during the exercise session and it involves dynamic movements or stretches. Doing a cool down facilitates the recovery of the body to a near-resting state post exercise and may involve flexibility exercises such as stretching.

3) Patient education

- Patient education helps to explain the pathophysiology, management strategies and the importance of compliance to the treatment. A general outline comparing the topics of patient education for cardiac and pulmonary conditions are listed below in Table 4. (Lung Foundation Australia: Pulmonary Rehabilitation Toolkit (https://pulmonaryrehab.com.au/))

Table 4. Main suggested educational topics for cardiac and pulmonary rehabilitation.

Type of advice	Cardiac rehabilitation	Pulmonary rehabilitation	General fitness
Exercise	Advice on physical activity and exercise prescription		
Pathophysiology and treatment	Information on disease Information on risk factors and management	Information on disease Role and correct use of medications (e.g. inhaler technique)	Information on risk factors and management
Management	Cardiovascular risk reduction Nutrition/healthy eating Stress management	Managing breathlessness Nutrition/diet management Energy conservation/ pacing Coping and management of depression, anxiety, and panic attacks	Cardiovascular risk reduction Nutrition/healthy eating Falls prevention (if applicable)
Smoking cessation	Yes, if required		

4) Program evaluation

An evaluation should be offered after patients have completed the rehabilitation program. Evaluation of the effectiveness of the program can be based on patient outcomes such as fitness, quality of life and confidence for self-management, as well as patient feedback on the general structure/content of the program.

5) Maintenance

Maintenance programs are to ensure that improvements in exercise capacity and self-management practices are continued. Some programs/activities may include: maintenance or booster exercise programs in the community, support groups, or regular reviews and reassessments.

Case studies

Case 1

Mr. Lee is a 60-year-old banker. He is a lifelong smoker who has been recently diagnosed with mild chronic obstructive pulmonary disease. He is currently still smoking 1 packet of cigarettes a day and is keen to stop. He has no other significant medical history and does not exercise regularly. He tends to get breathless when he has to climb stairs or walk longer distances of 1 km to the mass rapid transit station and needs to stop for a break.

Lifestyle changes/education:

- Smoking cessation
- Inhaler technique and compliance
    - He may be starting on new inhalers and therefore may benefit from education of proper usage techniques and the uses of different inhalers
- Breathlessness techniques
    - He may start to complain about breathlessness with activity/exertion and therefore may benefit with education of breathing techniques such as purse-lip breathing and positioning and to help him to understand the mechanism of how and why he gets breathless
- Regular exercise and activity
- Pathophysiology of chronic obstructive pulmonary disease (COPD)
    - As the diagnosis is new, he may benefit from education of the pathophysiology of COPD and its prognosis, treatment options and therefore hoping to increase compliance with treatment as well

Exercise prescription:

Endurance exercise

- Frequency: 3–5 times a week
- Intensity: BORG 3–4 on the Modified BORG Dyspnea scale (Table 3)
- Time: 20–30 minutes, not including warm up/cool down
- Type: walking, cycling

Strengthening Exercise

- Frequency: 3–5 times a week
- Intensity: BORG 3–4 on the Modified BORG Dyspnea scale (Table 3)
- Time: About 10 repetitions, 3 sets, type/equipment: dumbbells/body weight

Case 2

Mdm. Ling is a 50-year-old lady who has been recently discharged from hospital for an acute myocardial infarction. She has single vessel disease that was stented and has completed her short stint of cardiac rehabilitation program. She is now keen to continue exercises to improve her cardiovascular fitness. She has also recently been diagnosed with hyperlipidemia.

Lifestyle changes/education:

- Healthy eating and dietary modifications
  - ▪ She is newly diagnosed with hyperlipidemia and would benefit from reinforcement on the healthy diet choices to reduce her bad cholesterol
  - ▪ Reduce salt in diet, season with spices and herbs instead
  - ▪ Snack on fruits and vegetables instead of processed foods like deep fried food, biscuits, salty snacks, cakes, and pastries
  - ▪ Switch carbohydrates to whole grains (e.g. whole meal bread, brown rice)
  - ▪ Modify cooking styles to include more boiling, steaming, baking, roasting, and grilling, rather than deep frying
  - ▪ Replace cooking oils to polyunsaturated fat oils such as canola, soybean, corn, and olive oil
  - ▪ Limit alcohol: 1 standard drink = 20 g of alcohol/⅔ can (220 ml) of beer/1 glass (100 ml) of wine/1 nip (30 ml) of spirit
    - Women: 2 standard drinks/day
    - Men: 3 standard drinks/day
- Medication compliance
  - o She will benefit from reinforcement on medication counselling as she will be on long-term blood thinners, statins for her high cholesterol, and other medications
- Regular exercise and activity
- Stress management
  - o She will benefit from counselling on managing a good healthy lifestyle and reducing stress

Exercise prescription:

- Frequency: 3–5 times a week
- Intensity: 40–60% of heart rate reserve using the Karvonen formula gradually progressing to higher intensity
- Time: 30 minutes to accumulate to 150 minutes per week of exercise, not including warm up/cool down
- Type:
  - Endurance: walking, cycling, swimming, stair climbing
  - Strengthening: using free weights, dumbbells, resistance bands, machines

When to refer patients to a cardiac, pulmonary, or rehabilitation medicine specialist?

A patient may require closer monitoring or supervision for their exercise program, therefore a referral to a healthcare professional may be encouraged in the following situations:

1) Homebound or is a limited community ambulator due to breathlessness, fatigue, and/or deconditioning
2) Symptomatic or have increased breathlessness on daily activities/walking
3) On long-term oxygen therapy
4) Having significant musculoskeletal pain
5) High risk: pulmonary hypertension, implanted cardiac devices, untreated cardiovascular lesions, poorly controlled heart failure, poorly controlled comorbidities, poor insight

Recommended reading

- Garvey C, Bayles MP *et al.* Pulmonary rehabilitation exercise prescription in chronic obstructive pulmonary disease: review of selected guidelines: an official statement from the American Association of Cardiovascular and Pulmonary Rehabilitation. *J Cardiopulm Rehabil Prev.* 2016;36(2):75–83.

- Liguori G. *ACSM's guidelines for exercise testing and prescription, 11th edition.* Philadelphia: Lippincott Williams & Wilkins (2021), ISBN: 9781975150181 (spiral bound).
- Measuring physical activity intensity. *CDC.* 2022. Retrieved from https://www.cdc.gov/physicalactivity/basics/measuring/index.html
- Pulmonary rehabilitation toolkit. (n.d.). *Lung Foundation Australia.* Retrieved March 27, 2023. Retrieved from https://lungfoundation.com.au/health-professionals/clinical-information/pulmonary-rehabilitation/pr-toolkit/

- **QR Codes for Patient Education:**

Exercise: Carers X Physios (TTSH)

Diet/Healthy Living Advice (HealthHub)

Smoking Cessation (HealthHub)

Cardiac Rehabilitation Educational Videos

9

Rehabilitation of Chronic Musculoskeletal Pain

KIM Jong Moon, YAP Eng Ching

Introduction

This chapter on chronic musculoskeletal pain is divided by anatomical region into 3 main sections: spine, upper, and lower limbs. Clinical vignettes are presented followed by questions and answers covering history and physical examination, investigations, and diagnoses to management and rehabilitation to optimise function.

Definition of pain

The International Association for Study of Pain (IASP) defined pain as an unpleasant sensation with a subjective bio-psycho-social experience. It is secondary to an actual or potential tissue damage and is often associated with adverse impact on function.

How common is chronic pain?

Chronic pain is persistent pain over 3 to 6-month duration. About 20% of the world population are affected by chronic pain. It is more common in females and with increasing age. Majority of chronic pain affects the musculoskeletal system; lower back is the most common site. In 2017, the point prevalence of back pain was about 7.5% of global population.

Nociceptive pain

In a normal somatosensory nervous system, nociceptive pain occurs when a noxious stimulus causes a potential or an actual non-neural tissue damage, and manifests as a localised aching dull sore or throbbing pain.

Neuropathic pain

Neuropathic pain, on the other hand, occurs in a malfunctioning somatosensory system in the presence or absence of a noxious or non-noxious stimulus. Clinically the pain may be described as burning, cutting, electrical, stabbing, or tingling. Other features of neuropathic pain include allodynia and/or hyperalgesia. Allodynia is a phenomenon when a stimulus that is normally not painful (e.g. light touch) triggers pain. Hyperalgesia is a phenomenon when a mildly painful stimulus triggers severe pain, i.e. there is increased pain sensitivity.

Chronic pain sensitisation

Sensitization is a phenomenon of chronic pain when there is a reduced threshold and/or an increased pain response. Clinical manifestations include allodynia and hyperalgesia. This phenomenon in the peripheral or central nervous system is termed peripheral or central sensitisation respectively.

How can the patient subjectively rate neck and back pain intensity?

Patient could subjectively rate her pain intensity by using the numerical rating scale from 0 to 10 (0 is no pain and 10 is worst possible pain). The Wong-Baker faces pain rating scale with a series of 6 faces from happy face (0) to crying face (10) helps patient communicate pain intensity using the chart of facial expressions that best correspond to her pain intensity.

Three phases of soft-tissue healing after tissue injury

The first phase of soft-tissue healing is the cellular response to injury. The second phase includes the repair and regeneration, and the third phase is scar remodelling. Characteristics of chronic injuries are less intense inflammation, progressive functional impairments, and a tendency toward reinjury. Advanced age is also associated with decreased collagen synthesis and impaired tendon healing.

Rehabilitation of chronic neck and low back pain

A 60-year-old lady complained of chronic neck and back pain for 6 months. There was no history of trauma. She also had headache and dizziness when the neck ache was severe. Recently, the pain had spread down the outer aspects of her right upper and lower limbs.

Where are the pain generators in chronic neck and back pain?

Chronic neck and back pain predominantly arise from soft tissues: muscles and ligaments. Chronic pain may also arise from nerves, bones, and joints. Mechanical pain, also known as vertebral dysfunction, is a common cause of back and neck pain. Psychologic overlays: emotions and poor sleep also frequently contribute to chronic pain.

How spine movements affect the biomechanical pain generators in chronic neck and back pain

A functional unit of the spine comprises 2 adjacent vertebrae. A motion unit comprises a 3 joint complex: a large intervertebral joint anteriorly and a pair of small facet/zygapophyseal joints between the articular processes posteriorly.

a. During forward flexion

- The cross sectional area of lumbar canal increases and stenotic symptoms may be relieved
- Anterior elements of the spine which include the vertebral body and intervertebral disc, are loaded and stressed. Symptoms from these pain generators can be aggravated

b. During extension

- The cross sectional area of lumbar canal decreases, stenotic symptoms can be aggravated
- Posterior elements of the spine which include the facet joint and pars body, are loaded and stressed. Symptoms from these pain generators can be aggravated

c. Extension and ipsilateral flexion

- This narrows the neural foramen and radicular pain can be aggravated

d. Flexion and contra-lateral flexion

- Opens the neural foramen and radicular pain can be relieved

How different postures affect the biomechanical pain generator and back pain

If baseline of lumbar disc pressure when standing is 100%:

- The pressure increases to almost 150% when patient bends forward and when patient sits down; lumbar disc pain can be aggravated with these postures

- The pressure decreases to 25% when patient lies supine; lumbar disc pain may improve

Common pattern of muscle dysfunction in chronic neck and back pain

Neck and back muscles can be broadly divided into two groups: superficial global muscles responsible for trunk movement and deep local muscles responsible for trunk stabilisation.

In chronic neck and back pain:

- Superficial global muscles such as upper trapezius, scalenes, quadratus lumborum, and erector spinae tend to become overactive, hypertonic and tight
- Deep local muscles such as deep cervical flexors, multifidus, transversus abdominus, and pelvic floor muscles tend to become underactive, hypotonic, and lax

This imbalance of lax and tight muscles often leads to dysfunction. As the musculoskeletal system is a dynamic and inter-related kinetic chain, this dysfunction could cause ripple effects on proximal and distal musculoskeletal segments in the kinetic chain and a cascade of degeneration with clinical problems.

Main points to look for when taking history from the patient

Neck and back pain can be broadly divided into two main patterns of pain distribution: axial pain and radicular pain.

In addition, note the pain characteristics and intensity, nature of pain onset, any associated aggravating and relieving factor, whether pain is improving or worsening over time, impact on daily activities and any response to past treatment. Also look out for red flags and yellow flags of neck and back pain (see below).

Red flags of back and neck pain

They are signs and symptoms of sinister pathology:

- History of trauma
- Nocturnal pain, constant pain unresponsive to treatment
- Neurologic deficits such as extremity weakness
- Signs and symptoms of cauda equina syndrome (CES): saddle or bilateral lower limb signs or symptoms; bladder, bowel, or sexual dysfunction.

Urinary retention is the most common complaint in CES and is a surgical emergency

- Associated systemic symptoms such as fever, weight loss

Yellow flags of back and neck pain

They are psycho-social factors that indicate risk of long-term functional disability:

- Effect: low mood, anxiety, depression
- Beliefs and attitudes: catastrophizing and thinking the worst of pain symptoms, belief that pain and activity are harmful, and pain has to be eliminated before returning to normal activities
- Behaviour: fear and avoidance of activities, passive participation in rehabilitation and focus on passive modalities, sickness behaviour
- Work issues: unsupportive work environment, poor job satisfaction, pending claims, or compensations
- Social problems: social withdrawal, lack of social support, overprotective family, history of physical, or substance abuse

More objective way to quantify pain threshold and monitor progress (other than self-rated pain intensity score)

An algometer is a small handheld device that measures pressure pain threshold. Manual pressure is applied through its tip which is placed on a painful area. The pressure-pain threshold is the applied pressure when pain is experienced.

Approaching physical examination (PE) of the patient after history taking

One approach is to have a broad overview of the musculoskeletal system before narrowing down.

Look and move

- Look and inspect for obvious asymmetry or abnormality
- Move: examine for movement dysfunctions, active and passive range of motion, execution of functional movement of daily activities and gait

In the movement and screening examination, both quality and quantity of motion are noted. They provide clinical information to regions that may require further evaluation.

Feel and palpate

- Examine the muscles: core muscles for laxity and functional weakness, global muscles (eg erector spinae, quadratus lumborum) for hypertonicity and tenderness)
- Examine and exclude neurological deficits in the extremities

Tests for sacroiliac joint (SIJ) dysfunctions

- Gillet test: patient stands and raises one leg to 90 degrees. Ipsilateral posterior superior iliac spine (PSIS) should rotate inferiorly. Restriction of this motion is considered abnormal
- Seated flexion test: patient sits and bends forward. Asymmetric cephalad motion of PSIS indicates SIJ dysfunction
- FABER test: Flexion, Abduction and External Rotation (FABER) of the hip produces pain in dysfunctional SIJ
- Gaenslen's test: patient lies supine, flexes contralateral hip and drops leg off the bedside produces SIJ pain
- Iliac compression test: patient lies on side, downward force on iliac crest produces SIJ pain
- Yeoman's test: patient lies prone, hip extension and ilium rotation produce SIJ pain

How to clinically test the patient's core muscle function?

Core stabilisers are deep muscles and often not amenable to palpation. There are clinical tests to examine the function of core stabilisers.

- Straight leg lowering test: when patient lies supine with unilateral straight leg raised, the raised lower limb is lowered gradually down to the couch while keeping lumbar spine down on the examiner's hand sandwiched between the lumbar spine and couch. Patient with strong core stabilizers can lower the lower limb to a lower level before lumbar spine lifts from examiner's hand and curves away from the couch. The strength of core stabilizers could also be tested indirectly by asking patient to keep the lower limb raised at about 20 degrees from the couch against resistance
- Pelvic stabilisation and bridge test: when patient lies supine with knees flexed, the buttock is slowly lifted from couch while keeping the pelvis balanced (i.e. neutral and not tilted to either side). Difficulty of this test can

be increased with single leg bridge (i.e. bridge with unilateral straight leg raised at mid-range). Clinician can also add pressure resistance on either side of the pelvis. In a younger patient, the difficulty can be further increased with single leg stand and squat test while keeping the pelvis balanced

Clinical tests to determine if the patient has back pain from lumbar nerve tension

Clinical tests that increase lumbar neural tension may reproduce or exacerbate these back pain symptoms.

- Lasegue straight leg raise: sciatic pain when hip is flexed with knee extended, the pain is relieved by knee flexion and aggravated by foot dorsiflexion
- Bowstring: when straight leg raise elicits sciatica, flex knee to reduce symptom and then apply pressure on popliteal fossa to reproduce symptom
- Slump test: when patient is seated with neck flexed, spine is slumped forward with straight leg raised and ankle dorsi-flexed, radiating sciatic pain is reproduced or exacerbated. The symptom is relieved by reversing the manoeuvre
- Crossed straight leg raise: sciatic pain down the contralateral lower limb is a sign of severe nerve root impingement
- Femoral stretch/reverse lasegue straight leg raise: patient lies prone and examiner passively extends hip with knee flexed to 90 degrees. Pain down the anterior lateral thigh is a sign of femoral nerve root tension

Neural tension tests of the upper limb

These clinical tests increase nerve tension in the upper limb to reproduce symptoms and radicular neck pain.

- Median nerve neural tension: this manoeuvre comprises ipsilateral shoulder abduction about 110 degrees with external rotation, forearm supination, wrist and finger extension, elbow extension with contralateral neck flexion (Figure 1)

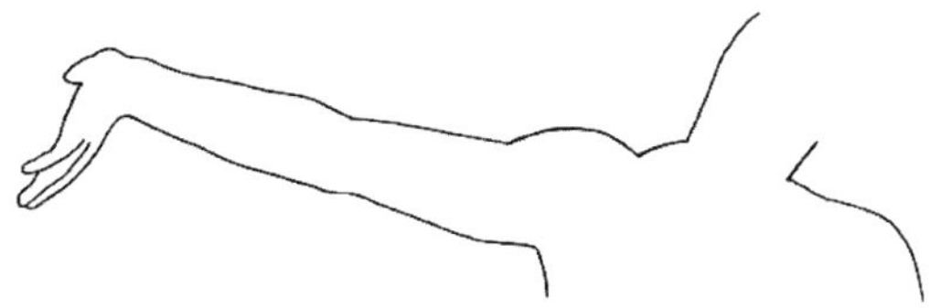

Figure 1. Median nerve neural tension.

- Radial nerve neural tension: this manoeuvre comprises ipsilateral shoulder abduction about 30 degrees with internal rotation, forearm pronation, wrist and finger flexion, elbow extension with contralateral neck flexion (Figure 2)
- Ulnar nerve neural tension: this manoeuvre comprises ipsilateral shoulder abduction about 90 degrees with external rotation, forearm supination wrist and fingers extension, elbow flexion with contralateral neck flexion (Figure 3)

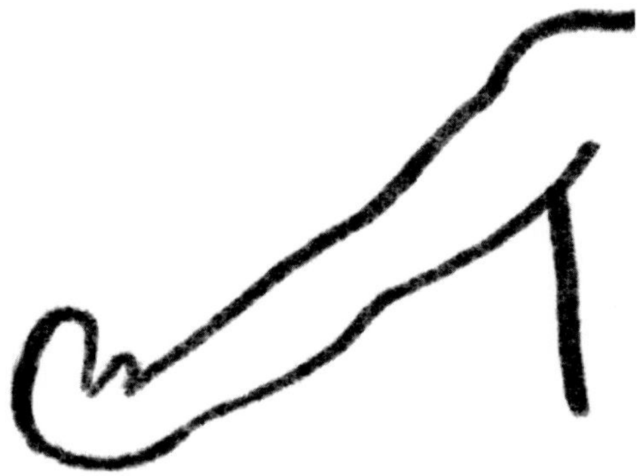

Figure 2. Radial nerve neural tension.

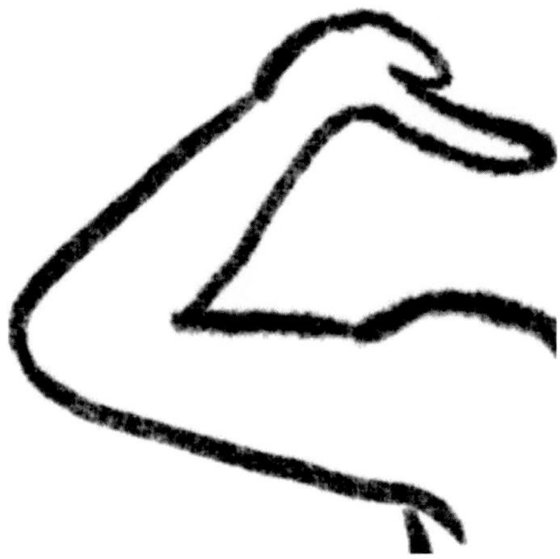

Figure 3. Ulnar nerve neural tension.

What other clinical tests may increase/relieve cervical neve tension or radicular neck pain?

- Increase cervical nerve tension or radicular symptoms
  a. Spurling's test — patient's neck is passively moved into ipsilateral flexion and extension, gentle downward axial compression is applied to reproduce radicular symptoms
  b. Valsalva manoeuvre — while sitting, patient takes a deep breath and holds the breath with forced exhalation against resistance to increase intra-spinal pressure and reproduce radicular symptoms
- Relieve cervical nerve tension or radicular symptoms
  a. Neck traction distraction test to open foramen and relieve radicular symptoms
  b. Shoulder abduction test — ipsilateral palm is placed on top of head to relieve nerve tension and radicular symptoms

Double crush syndrome

It is a syndrome when peripheral nerve compressions occur at 2 locations along its course. Peripheral nerve compression at one location may predispose it to injury at another location. Symptomatic threshold of compression at the second location is decreased and the cumulated intensity of symptoms of concomitant compressions is increased. A common double crush syndrome in the upper limb is cervical 6 radiculopathy with carpal tunnel syndrome. Patient may complain of numbness and pain over the lateral aspect of upper limb, palm, and neck. The diagnoses can be evaluated anatomically with imaging tests and electro-physiologically with electro-diagnostic study i.e. nerve conduction test and electromyography.

Can neck pain cause headache?

Cervicogenic headache is a type of chronic headache arising from cervico-occipital and/or upper cervical joint dysfunction. The headache is usually unilateral. The pain may spread proximally from occiput to frontal areas and/or distally to shoulder and arm. Cervicogenic headache improves with treatment targeted at the underlying cervical dysfunction.

Can neck pain cause dizziness?

Dizziness is a symptom frequently associated with neck pain. Afferent proprioceptive endings commonly found in cervical soft tissues are closely connected with visual and vestibular centres. Cervical dysfunction disrupts this proprioceptive equilibrium and causes sensation of imbalance. Cervicogenic dizziness is a diagnosis of exclusion. Treatment directed at underlying cervical dysfunction improves the dizziness.

Waddell signs

They are signs of non-organic back pain:

1. Sensitive and tender back pain on light superficial palpation
2. Non-anatomic sensory/motor abnormalities, widespread pain
3. Simulation tests:
   - Low back pain on cranial axial loading
   - Back pain on shoulder-pelvic rotation
4. Distraction tests: straight leg raise test when patient is supine and when patient is seated
5. Over-reaction to testing and examination

Further investigations of the patient

In the absence of red flags, it is reasonable to initially manage most cases of neck and back pain without further investigation. Imaging studies reveal static anatomic findings. Electro-diagnostic studies reveal dynamic physiology of muscle and nerve function. Over 25% of asymptomatic population have abnormal findings and degeneration on their MRI spine. The prevalence of abnormal imaging rises with increasing age. Abnormal findings on imaging scan may not be the source of pain. Clinicians must correlate the history with physical examination, test findings and treatment response to determine the likely pain generator. Imaging guided injection procedure may provide further diagnostic information on the likely pain generator, as well as therapeutic benefit to augment progress of rehabilitation and improve function.

Approaching management of chronic neck and back pain in the patient

In the absence of red flags, majority of back pain and neck pain can be managed conservatively. It is important to explain pain and help patient understand why the neck and back hurt to assist self-management and improve daily function.

Absolute rest leads to deconditioning and functional decline. Relative rest with graduated resumption of functional activities are more appropriate. The signs and symptoms of neurological dysfunction are not always due to anatomical nerve root compression. It can be due to nerve root irritation and inflammation. Muscle imbalance and dysfunction can also contribute to neurological complaints and symptoms.

The goal of rehabilitation is not to cure pain. The aim is to help reduce pain intensity and frequency, enable self-management, and improve daily function.

Role of physical modalities in management of chronic neck and back pain

Physical modalities such as traction, heat, and electrical therapy, if not contraindicated, may help as supplementary treatment of chronic neck and back pain. However, they are passive therapeutic modalities, and their effects are usually temporary. Braces and corsets may also help as short-term adjunctive treatment. Deconditioning could result from prolonged use.

Prescription of back exercises in the management of chronic back pain

- Extension biased back exercises are often prescribed if back pain arises from anterior elements of the lumbar spine — inter-vertebral disc or vertebral body
- Flexion biased back exercises are often prescribed if back pain arises from posterior elements of the lumbar spine — facet joint or pars body
- Active conditioning, core, and gluteal exercises help to rebalance back muscles and yield improved long-term outcome

Neural Mobilization exercises to manage radicular neck and back pain

When the patient has radicular neck pain from cervical 6 +/− median nerve irritation at carpal tunnel, we can modify the median nerve neural tension test described earlier by alternately decreasing and increasing neural tension proximally and distally (i.e. coupling ipsilateral neck flexion proximally with wrist-finger extension distally, then coupling contralateral neck flexion proximally with wrist-finger flexion distally) to glide and mobilise the affected nerve along its course.

When the patient has radicular back pain, we can modify the neural tension slump test described earlier by alternately decreasing and increasing neural tension proximally and distally (i.e. coupling neck extension proximally with straight leg raise and ankle dorsiflexion distally, then coupling neck flexion proximally with knee flexion and ankle plantar flexion distally) to glide the affected lumbar-sacral nerve along its course. (Figure 4)

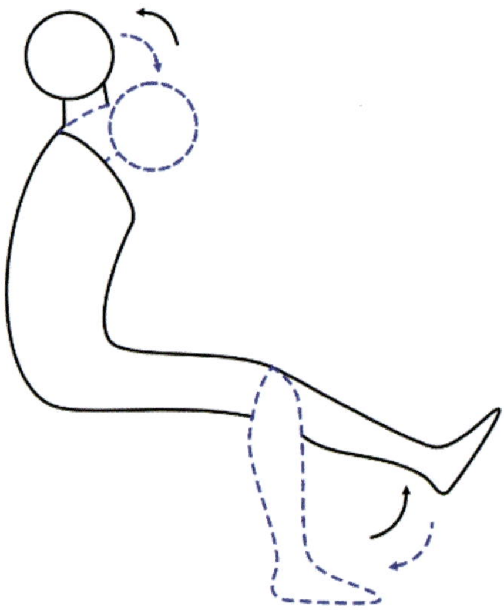

Figure 4. Modify neural tension slump test for neural mobilization.

Prescription of medications in the management of chronic neck and back pain

- Analgesics help to control neck and back pain, reduce inflammation, and dampen sensitisation. Commonly used analgesics include paracetamol, non-steroidal anti-inflammatory drugs, and synthetic opiate analogue such as tramadol
- Adjuvant analgesics: anticonvulsants such as gabapentin and pregabalin dampen central sensitisation, antidepressants such as tricyclics (e.g. amitriptyline, nortriptyline) and serotonin-norepinephrine reuptake inhibitor (e.g. duloxetine) enhance central descending inhibition of neuropathic pain
- Adjuvants and analgesics with attendant somnolent effect also help improve sleep and relieve muscle fatigue

Interdisciplinary biopsychosocial approach to chronic back and neck pain management

Chronic back and neck pain patients often present with de-conditioning and psychosocial issues with multiple barriers to recovery. Such patients will benefit from a comprehensive interdisciplinary rehabilitation approach, biomedical management together with an active conditioning exercise program coupled with cognitive behavioural therapy to enable self-management and optimise function.

Prognosis of neck and back pain

After an acute episode of neck pain, majority of patients will improve with or without treatment. However, about 50% will continue to suffer frequent recurrences or residual pain. Low back dysfunction often persists even when the pain has resolved. 90% of back pain subsides within 3 months. However, 80% of cases continue to have recurrent pain in the subsequent 1 to 2 years. About 10% suffer chronic residual symptoms.

Rehabilitation of upper limb pain

Shoulder pain

A 53-year-female complains of right shoulder pain and limited range of motion for 1 month. She denies any previous shoulder injury, upper limb fracture, or chest surgery. She has difficulty in reaching for car's seat belt and fastening her bra. Her pain is aggravated by right lateral decubitus position.

Main difference in physical examination of shoulder range of motion between adhesive capsulitis and rotator cuff tear

There is a reduction in both passive and active shoulder range of motion, particularly at external rotation and abduction in adhesive capsulitis. In rotator cuff tears, active range of motion is restricted but passive range of motion may normal.

Clinical tests for shoulder impingement

- Neer's test is positive if pain is reproduced with forward flexion of the arm in internal rotation
- Hawkins-Kennedy test is positive if there is pain with forward flexion of the humerus to 90 degrees with forcible internal rotation of the shoulder
- Yocum test is positive if there is pain with raising the elbow while the ipsilateral hand is on the contralateral shoulder
- Painful arc test is positive if there is pain with shoulder elevation between 60 and 120 degrees

Three stages of adhesive capsulitis

In stage 1, the painful stage or the freezing stage, the gradual onset of progressive pain is worse during the night and exacerbated by overhead activities. The patients gradually report a loss of motion. In stage 2, the frozen stage or the adhesive stage, there is a gradual decrease in pain, but this stage is associated with a reduction in the range of motion and decreased use of the affected shoulder. Stage 3, the thawing stage, is characterised by a gradual decrease in pain and increase in the pain-free range of motion.

Conservative management of adhesive capsulitis

Conservative management includes physical modalities, analgesics, activity modification, intraarticular corticosteroid injection, postural retraining, and ROM exercises. For patients who do not improve after 6 months of conservative management, more aggressive treatments such as capsular hydrodilatation, manipulation under anaesthesia, and arthroscopic lysis of adhesion can be considered.

Non-operative treatment of rotator cuff tendinopathy

During the acute stage of rehabilitation, controlling pain and inflammation is important. Physical therapy treatment consists of soft tissue mobilisation, passive range of motion, and joint stabilisation. In recovery stage of rehabilitation, restoring range of motion to the shoulder complex by active assisted range of motion exercises can be started. Strengthening of the scapular muscles and rotator cuff musculature should be started during this phase. Advanced strengthening of rotator cuff and the scapular stabilizers should be the focus during the functional stages of rehabilitation. In addition, proprioceptive training and functional rehabilitation can be started during this phase.

Elbow pain

A 42-year-male complains of right lateral elbow pain for 2 months after playing tennis. On physical examination, left upper limb sensory examination is normal but motor power of wrist and finger extensor is slightly diminished. Cozen test is positive. Elbow range of motion is within normal range.

Cozen test and its clinical significance

In Cozen test, the patient is asked to fully extend the elbow, pronate the forearm, and make a fist. The examiner then resists the patient's attempt to extend and radially deviate the wrist. This test is positive if pain develops over the lateral aspect of the elbow. Positive Cozen test suggests lateral epicondylitis.

Main pathologic change of lateral epicondylitis and most commonly affected muscle

The main pathologic change of lateral epicondylitis is degenerative change (angiofibroblastic hyperplasia). The degenerative changes occur most commonly in the origin of the extensor carpi radialis brevis.

Non-operative treatment for lateral epicondylitis

Non-operative treatment includes avoidance of provocative activities, oral analgesics, physical modalities, bracing (counterforce brace or neutral wrist splint), equipment modification (reducing string tension and enlarging the grip size of tennis racket), stretching and strengthening exercise, corticosteroid injection, prolotherapy, platelet-rich plasma injection, autologous blood injection, and extracorporeal shock wave therapy.

Hand pain

A 61-year-old female complains of paraesthesia and numbness of right 1st to 4th fingertips for 1 month which is worse during the night. She also complains of intermittent right upper limb radiating pain.

Differential diagnosis

The differential diagnosis includes carpal tunnel syndrome (CTS), C6-7 radiculopathy, brachial plexopathy, proximal median neuropathy, Raynaud's phenomenon, generalised neuropathy, and arthritis of carpometacarpal joint of thumb.

Special provocation tests for carpal tunnel syndrome (CTS)

The common special tests for CTS include the:

- Phalen test
- Tinel test
- Reverse Phalen test (wrist extension test)
- Carpal compression test

Electrodiagnostic findings of the wrist

The electrodiagnostic findings of focal demyelination of median nerve at the wrist include conduction velocity slowing across wrist and prolonged distal latency of median motor & sensory nerve.

Ultrasonographic findings of CTS

Ultrasonographic findings of CTS include the enlargement of the median nerve at the carpal tunnel inlet (scaphoid-pisiform level), the flattening of median nerve at the flexor retinaculum level (at the level of the hook of hamate), the palmar bowing of the flexor retinaculum, and the hypoechoic change & the altered fascicular change of median nerve.

Indication of surgical decompression of CTS

Indications of surgical decompression include severe wasting and weakness of the thumb abductor, persistent numbness, or paresthesia, failed conservative measures, ongoing denervation in abductor pollicis brevis on needle EMG and presence of a mass lesion.

Rehabilitation of lower limp pain

Groin pain

A 73-year-male complains of right groin pain and stiffness for 6 months. He denies any previous hip injury or disease. His pain is worse with weight bearing or walking. His pain is relieved with rest. Sometime his groin pain radiates to medial knee.

Common antalgic gait patterns

Antalgic gait patterns from unilateral disease are characterised by decreased single-limb stance time on the painful limb, shortened stride length for the contralateral limb, increased double support time, and slowed walking speed.

Positive FABER manoeuvre (Patrick test) physical examination. What is your differential diagnosis?

The Flexion Abduction External Rotation (FABER) test is commonly utilised as a provocation test to detect hip or sacroiliac joint pathology. The differential diagnosis includes hip osteoarthritis, avascular necrosis of the femoral head, hip labral tear, hip joint infection, inflammatory arthropathy, protrusio acetabuli, acetabular fracture, or sacroiliac disease.

Typical radiographic findings of hip osteoarthritis

The typical radiographic findings of hip osteoarthritis are joint space narrowing, osteophyte, subchondral sclerosis, and subchondral cyst.

The patient was transferred to rehabilitation medicine after right total hip replacement with posterior approach.

Possible complications after surgery

The possible complications after posterior approach hip replacement includes deep vein thrombosis, dislocation of hip, wound or prosthetic joint infection, heterotopic ossification, aseptic loosening of the prosthesis, and sciatic nerve injury.

Hip precautions to observe in this patient

Standard precautions for a posterior approach are not flexing hip past 90 degrees, not adducting hip past midline, and not internally rotating hip past neutral.

When you review him 1 month after total hip replacement, he wants to drive his car and resume sports activities. What is your advice?

Driving until 8 weeks after joint replacement of right lower limb is not advisable because right lower limb braking reaction time is prolonged until 8 weeks after surgery. He will be able to resume low-impact sports such as swimming, cycling, golf, or walking between 3 and 6 months after surgery.

Lateral hip pain

A 45-year-old-female complains of left lateral hip pain radiating to the lateral aspect of the thigh for 2 months since starting golf lesson. She denies any direct contusion or trauma and does not have any significant past medical history. Pain is provoked by walking and running, particularly when the is in external rotation and abduction.

Differential diagnosis

The differential diagnosis of lateral hip pain includes greater trochanteric pain syndrome, lumbosacral radiculopathy, iliotibial band syndrome, osteoarthritis of the hip, avascular necrosis of the femoral head, leg length discrepancy, myofascial pain, heterotopic ossification, or acetabular labral disease.

Greater trochanteric pain syndrome (GTPS)

Greater trochanteric pain syndrome (GTPS) is a clinical diagnosis of lateral hip pain and includes gluteus medius tendinopathy or tear, gluteus minimus tendinopathy or tear, trochanteric bursitis, and external coxa saltans (snapping hip syndrome).

Contributing factors of GTPS

Several contributing factors have been associated with GTPS, including hip or knee osteoarthritis, lumbar spine degenerative disorders, obesity, leg length discrepancy (true or functional), iliotibial band tightness, and gait abnormalities.

Typical physical examination findings of GTPS

On physical examination of GTPS, localized tenderness is found on palpation of the greater trochanter. Lateral hip pain may be elicited with resisted hip abduction in side-lying position. Lateral hip pain may be aggravated by active hip internal or external rotation at 45 degrees of hip flexion.

Conservative management of GTPS

Conservative management options include analgesic or anti-inflammatory medication, sports, and activity modification (avoidance of exacerbating activities), stretching exercise of the iliotibial band, tensor fascia lata and gluteal muscles, strengthening exercise of hip abductors, extensors, and external rotators, local corticosteroid injection, PRP injection, and extracorporeal shock wave therapy.

Lateral knee pain

A 40-year-old male complains of right lateral knee sharp pain during running. Knee pain increases on downhill running. He denies any previous major knee injury or morning stiffness. On physical examination, joint instability and meniscus tests are negative. Joint swelling and warmth are not detected.

Differential diagnosis

Differential diagnosis of lateral knee in active individuals includes iliotibial band syndrome, patellofemoral pain syndrome, lateral meniscus tear, popliteus tendinitis, lateral collateral ligament injury, lateral hamstring strain, lumbar radiculopathy, common peroneal nerve injury, and distal femur bone stress injury.

Clinical tests for diagnosing iliotibial band syndrome

The noble compression test is a clinical tool in evaluating iliotibial band (ITB) syndrome. This test is performed with the patient supine. The patient is asked to do active knee flexion and extension while the examiner compresses the lateral femoral epicondyle. The test result is positive if the patient complains of severe pain over the lateral femoral epicondyle at 30 degrees of flexion.

The Ober test evaluates a tight or contracted iliotibial band. With the patient side-lying, the knee is supported and flex to 90 degrees. The hip is then abducted and extended, and the knee support is released. Failure of the knee to adduct is indicates a positive test.

Possible contributing factors of ITBS

Iliotibial band syndrome (ITBS) is an overuse injury as a result of the distal ITB impingement over the lateral femoral condyle due to compression or friction. Several factors associated with the risk of IBTS include weakness of hip abductors, ITB tightness, excessive foot-ankle pronation and supination, training errors (rapid changes in training routine), leg length discrepancy, and increased prominence of the lateral femoral epicondyle.

Rehabilitation management of ITBS

Physical modalities such as ultrasound, phonophoresis, iontophoresis, low-level laser therapy, and electrical stimulation may be used to reduce early inflammation and pain. Stretching exercise of ITB, iliopsoas, quadriceps, and gastrocnemius-soleus and strengthening exercise of hip abductors and vastus medialis obliquus are recommended. Myofascial release and muscle massage may reduce tension in the connective tissue. Off-the-shelf or custom made semirigid foot orthoses for improving subtalar motion and the position of the tibia may also be considered. Corticosteroid injections at ITB can be considered if pain does not improve with a course of physiotherapy.

Topical adverse effects of corticosteroid injection at ITB

Topical adverse reactions to corticosteroid injection include a transient flare of pain, tendon rupture, osteonecrosis, infection, injection site hypopigmentation and subcutaneous fast atrophy.

Anterior knee pain

A 28-year-old female complains of insidious onset of bilateral anterior knee pain for 4 months. Knee pain increases on descending of stairs, prolonged sitting, or squatting. She denies any previous major knee injury or morning stiffness.

Differential diagnosis

Differential diagnosis of anterior knee pain includes patellofemoral pain syndrome, infrapatellar fat pad syndrome (Hoffa's syndrome), peripatellar bursitis, patellar tendonitis, quadriceps tendonitis, patellofemoral arthritis, meniscus lesion, synovial plica syndromes, Osgood-Schlatter disease, and osteochondritis dissecans.

Patellar tracking disorder and the possible causes

Patellar tracking disorder means that the patella shifts out of place during knee flexion or extension. Several biomechanical abnormalities can cause improper tracking of patella. Tight quadriceps can create abnormal forces on the retropatellar cartilage. Tight ITB may lead to patella to track laterally. Ineffective vastus medialis oblique is unable to oppose the lateral full of a tight ITB. Pes planus with tibial internal rotation positions the patella medially. Anteversion of the femoral neck associated with external rotation of the tibia and compensatory pronation at the foot can cause increased force at the patella. Ineffective eccentric function of the hip external rotators fails to control femoral internal rotation during running. Weak hip abductors increase load on the ITB.

Patellar grind test (Clarke sign)

Patellar grind test (Clarke's sign) is used to evaluate for patellofemoral joint dysfunction. With the patient supine and knee extended, the examiner pushes the patella downward and distally. The patient is instructed to contract the quadriceps muscle. Pain with movements of the patella or an inability to complete the test is indicative of patellofemoral dysfunction.

Exercise program for patellofemoral pain syndrome

Exercise program for patellofemoral pain syndrome include quadriceps (particularly VMO) strengthening, gluteal and core muscle strengthening, stretching tight structures (ITB, quadriceps, hamstrings, calf), and patellofemoral joint mobilisation.

McConnell taping and the proposed mechanisms of taping

McConnell taping involves applying rigid tape across the patella, pulling from lateral to medial. This helps to reduce excessive lateral pull on the patella when the knee bends and reduces irritation of the patellofemoral joint. It may also activate the vastus medialis oblique (VMO) muscle. Another mechanism of patellar taping is repositioning of patella within the femoral trochlea groove. This alters the patellofemoral joint contact load and joint reaction force, thereby reducing pain.

Orthotic managements of patellofemoral pain syndrome

Orthotic management options for patellofemoral pain syndrome are patellofemoral control brace and foot orthosis for patients with hyperpronated feet.

Knee injury

A 25-year-old man presented with a 5-day history of right knee pain, swelling, and feelings of instability after sustaining an injury to his right leg while playing soccer. His right leg was planted in a flexed position when it was forcefully kicked from the side.

Two most commonly injured ligaments of knee

The most commonly injured knee ligaments are the medial collateral ligament (MCL) and the anterior cruciate ligament (ACL).

Clinical tests for evaluating acute ACL injury

The key physical examination for ACL injury in the patient with an acute injury is Lachman test, in which an anterior force is applied to the tibia with the knee in 20–30 degrees of flexion. Another test is the pivot shift test, in which the examiner attempts to reproduce anterolateral instability by internally rotating the leg while applying a valgus stress to the knee as it is flexed.

Three stages of ligament sprains

Grade I sprains demonstrate negligible loss of structural integrity and minimal signs of inflammation. In grade II sprains, partial rupture of the ligament is associated with significant pain and inflammation. The tensile strength of the involved tissue is reduced after the functional recovery. Grade III injuries are associated with complete tear of the ligament, chronic instability, susceptibility to recurrent sprains, and impaired proprioception of the involved joint.

Conservative treatment options for grade 1–2 MCL sprain

Initial treatment consists of aggressive use of ice and elevation of leg. Early, gentle knee flexion and extension exercises are initiated in the first 1 to 2 weeks. A knee immobiliser may be used for 1 to 2 weeks. Gradual return to full activities as tolerated is progressed over 1 to 4 weeks, depending on the severity of the injury.

Closed kinetic chain exercises

Closed kinetic chain exercises are commonly prescribed in rehabilitation exercises. In closed kinetic chain exercise, the distal segment of the extremity is fixed, and the proximal segments are free to move. Closed kinetic chain exercises allow for the simultaneous activation of antagonistic muscle groups, thus promoting increased joint stability and a simulation of functional movement patterns.

Indications of surgical referral for ACL injury

In general, younger patients and those with a high activity level (high-demand on rotatory and lateral movement sports) should be considered for ACL reconstruction. When associated injuries are present, especially if these cause mechanical symptoms, surgical treatment should be considered.

Chronic ankle pain

A 35-year-old male complains of pain and swelling around the right lateral malleolus area after spraining his ankle, with the ankle inverted, 6 months ago. He had 2 similar episodes 1 and 3 years ago. On examination, mild weakness of right ankle eversion is noted. Sensory testing of right foot and ankle is normal.

Clinical tests for evaluating mechanical laxity of the ankle joint

Anterior drawer test is used to detect anterior talocrural joint laxity. The patient is supine or seated, knee flexed to 90 degrees, ankle plantar flexed 10–20 degrees. The examiner stabilizes the anterior distal leg with one hand and grasps the heel with the other hand and pulls the heel anteriorly. A positive test results if the talus translates forward.

Talar tilt test is used to examine the anterior talofibular ligament and calcaneofibular ligament. The patient is seated with 10–20 degrees of plantarflexion. The distal lower leg is stabilized with one hand and the hindfoot is inverted with the other hand. The lateral aspect of the talus is palpated to determine if tilting occurs. The degree of laxity is compared with the normal ankle.

Diagnostic imaging studies to confirm chronic ankle instability

Routine radiographs are useful to rule out old or chronic fractures, to assess the integrity of the ankle mortise, and to assess for ankle arthritis. Stress radiographs (anterior drawer, inversion stress) may be helpful in determining mechanical instability. CT and bone scans can identify subtle talus fractures, stress fracture, and other bone diseases. MRI and MR arthrography give the most information about soft tissue injury.

He is wearing an ankle support. When can this be weaned off?

The goal with ankle supports is to prevent recurrent sprains and further tissue trauma. Many patients can successfully be weaned from external supports after rehabilitation. However, high-demand athletes may choose to brace or to tape during athletic participation indefinitely.

Rehabilitation program of chronic ankle instability

Rehabilitation starts by restoring ankle dorsiflexion and eversion. Care must be taken to avoid recurrent inversion stress to the ankle. The patient begins an ankle muscle group strengthening program with an emphasis on ankle evertor strengthening. Strengthening may start with low-level submaximal isometric exercises, and progress in a pain-free dynamic and isokinetic strengthening. Balance and proprioceptive exercises have been found to decrease symptoms and the rate of re-injury. The devices for proprioceptive training are ankle disks and wobble boards. Functional exercises and sports-specific drills can begin when the patient has full range of motion, no pain, and at least 85% peroneal strength compared with the contralateral ankle.

Non-surgical interventional procedures for chronic ankle instability

Corticosteroid injection is not advised and may further weaken the ligaments. Prolotherapy can be considered. The injectate (low-concentration dextrose solution) acts as a local tissue irritant and induces ligament and capsular hypertrophy. Orthobiologic intervention such as platelet rich plasma can be considered for the interventional treatment of ankle ligament injury as well.

Recommended reading

- Cifu DX. *Braddom's physical medicine and rehabilitation, 6th edition.* Netherlands: Elsevier (2020).
- Frontera WR, Silver JK *et al. Essentials of physical medicine and rehabilitation, 4th edition.* Netherlands: Elsevier (2020).
- Haig A, Colwell M. *Back pain: a guide for the primary care physician.* United States: American College of Physicians Press (2005).
- International Association for the Study of Pain (IASP). Retrieved from https://www.iasp-pain.org
- Liebenson C. *Rehabilitation of the spine: a patient-centered approach, 3rd edition.* Netherlands: Wolters Kluwer (2019).
- Stout A. *Low back pain, an issue of physical medicine and rehabilitation clinics, 1st edition* (2010).

10

Intensive Care Rehabilitation

THAM Shuen-Loong, SENG Wai Ping Alfred

Introduction

Advances in critical care medicine have led to an improvement in the number of critical illness survivors in the last decade. However, some of these survivors develop affective disorders, physical, and/or cognitive dysfunction, stemming from their time in the Intensive Care Unit (ICU). This translates to a wave of patients requiring multidisciplinary rehabilitation, often for a protracted amount of time. Such disabilities may be persistent for years following discharge from ICU/ hospital, placing further economic burden on the patient, family, and community.

Case

Mr Tan was a 45-year-old male with hypertension, diabetes mellitus, asthma, and hyperlipidemia. He underwent saucerization of a large back carbuncle followed by a stormy intensive care unit (ICU) stay. He had ventilator- associated pneumonia and underwent prolonged intubation for 2 weeks. Despite successful extubation, he had persisting physical and cognitive dysfunction. He was discharged from hospital after 12 weeks, requiring physical assistance in some of his basic activities of daily living. At 1 year, he still remained unable to return to work (as a taxi driver) even though he was able to manage self-care independently at home. Since his ICU stay, he was diagnosed with unrelenting depressive and anxiety issues.

Post-intensive care syndrome (PICS)

Post-intensive care syndrome (PICS) is a collection of new or increased physical, cognitive, and mental health symptoms that occurs during the ICU stay and persists after a patient leaves the ICU. The family and caregivers can also experience new or increased mental health issues after a patient is hospitalised in a critical care setting. This is denoted as *post-intensive care syndrome–family* (PICS-F). Limited awareness related to PICS (and PICS-F), may lead to reduced quality of life and increased suffering for these patients and their families.

Burden of PICS

Various impairments can last for years in ICU survivors:

- New physical impairments ~25–80%
- Cognitive impairments ~30–80% of ICU survivors
- Psychiatric illnesses ~8–57% of patients
- Reduction in employment ~50% for ICU survivors at discharge who were gainfully employed pre-ICU
- Needing care assistance at 6 months post ICU-discharge: ~25%

1. Physical impairment

Critically ill patients frequently acquire muscle weakness whilst in the ICU. This is termed ICU-acquired weakness (ICUAW) and has a reported prevalence of 43%. Risk factors associated with ICUAW are listed in Table 1.

Several non-mutually exclusive pathophysiologic mechanisms are responsible for ICUAW:

- **Muscle atrophy:** catabolic state of critical illness, immobilisation/ denervation
- **Muscle dysfunction:** bioenergetic failure from mitochondrial damage, reduced autophagy, structural muscle alterations (replacement with adipose tissue and fibrosis), inflammation, necrosis from microcirculatory changes (impaired perfusion, oxygen delivery)
- **Denervation:** membrane and ion channel dysfunction lead to hypo or non-excitability of nerve and muscle

ICUAW can occur in the following ways, singly or in combination, leading to varied clinical presentations:

i. **Polyneuropathy** (also known as critical illness polyneuropathy) — characterised by a symmetrical, distal sensori-motor axonopathy, affecting limb and respiratory muscles

ii. **Myopathy** (also known as critical illness myopathy) — proximal muscles more affected than distal muscles; involving limb and respiratory muscles

iii. **Muscle atrophy**

Table 1. Risk factors implicated in ICUAW.

Non-modifiable risk factors		Modifiable risk factors	
• Demographics	Older age, female	• Hyperglycemia	
• Premorbid	Frail/multiple comorbidities, premorbid disability	• Parenteral nutrition	
• Severity of illness	Higher illness severity score, systemic inflammation/sepsis, multiorgan failure, high lactate level	• Drugs	Vasoactive medications (e.g. ß-agonist), antibiotics (e.g. vancomycin, aminoglycoside), sedatives, prolonged neuromuscular blockade, corticosteroids
		• Immobility	

Appendicular (peripheral), core, respiratory muscles and even muscles of swallowing may be affected. This will invariably result in impairment in activities of daily living performance (including self-care tasks like feeding, grooming, dressing, showering, and toileting), respiratory function, and oral intake.

Assessment of muscle function in ICUAW:

- Manual muscle testing
  The strength of pre-determined 6 muscle groups (wrist flexion, elbow flexion, shoulder abduction, ankle dorsiflexion, knee extension, and hip flexion) are tested in according to the Medical Research Council grades (MRC 0–5). Performed bilaterally, the highest possible score of 60 can be obtained. Significant weakness is seen in patients with a score less than 48. A score of less than 36 signifies severe weakness

- Electrophysiology studies
  Electromyography (EMG) and nerve conduction studies. These can differentiate between critical illness polyneuropathy and myopathy (Table 2)

- Muscle or nerve tissue pathology studies
  Biopsy of muscle and nerve (research tool)

- For respiratory muscle strength assessment
  Maximal inspiratory and expiratory pressure for global respiratory strength. Bedside ultrasonography of diaphragm: diaphragmatic excursion and thickness (for strength and atrophy)

Table 2. Electrophysiological and tissue pathology study findings in critical illness polyneuropathy and myopathy.

	Critical illness polyneuropathy	Critical illness myopathy
CMAP amplitude	Decreased	Decreased
CMAP duration	Normal	Increased
SNAP amplitude	Decreased	Normal
Nerve conduction velocity	Normal or near normal	Normal or near normal
EMG at rest	Fibrillation potentials/positive sharp waves	Fibrillation potentials/positive sharp waves
MUP voluntary muscle activation	Long duration, high amplitude, polyphasic	Short duration, low amplitude
Repetitive nerve stimulation	Absence of decremental response	Absence of decremental response
Direct muscle stimulation	Normal muscle excitability	Reduced muscle excitability
Nerve biopsy	Primary distal axonal degeneration, no demyelination	Normal
Muscle biopsy	Denervation atrophy of type 1 and 2 muscle fibres	A spectrum of abnormalities: myofiber atrophy, angulated fibres, necrosis, fatty degeneration, focal, or diffuse loss of thick filaments

(CMAP: Compound Muscle Action Potential, SNAP: Sensory Nerve Action Potential, MUP: Motor Unit Potential)

2. Cognitive impairment

Delirium is defined as a disturbance of consciousness with impaired attention, accompanied by a change in cognition or perceptual disturbance that develops over a short span of time and tends to fluctuate over the course of the day. Delirium in the ICU is a significant problem for critically ill patients. A prevalence of 31% was observed in this population.

Delirium subtypes:

- Hypoactive subtype (commonest): 17% (associated with a worse outcome)
- Mixed motor subtype: 10%
- Hyperactive: 4%

The patient with hypoactive delirium exhibits slowed mentation, lethargy, and decreased movement. This silent clinical nature makes it an easily overlooked entity in the ICU.

Delirium in critically ill patients is strongly associated with cognitive impairment after ICU discharge. ICU delirium is also associated with poor outcome, lengthier ICU and hospital length of stay (LOS), and cost. Rapidly reversible, sedation-related delirium, however, does not signify the same poor prognosis as persistent delirium.

Numerous risk factors for ICU delirium have been studied. Significant strong associations include benzodiazepine use, blood transfusions, greater age, dementia, prior coma, pre-ICU emergency surgery, or trauma and higher disease severity. (Table 3)

Table 3. Risk factors for ICU delirium.

Modifiable risk factors	Non-modifiable risk factors
Benzodiazepine use	Older age
Blood transfusions	Dementia
	Prior coma
	Pre-ICU emergency surgery or trauma
	Increasing APACHE (Acute Physiology and Chronic Health Evaluation) scores
	Increasing ASA (American Society of Anaesthesiologists) scores

Apart from delirium in ICU, ICU survivors could well experience problems related to processing speed, memory, attention, and executive functioning. In fact, a longer duration of delirium in the hospital was found to be associated with worse global cognition. Cognitive deficits can be persistent for years following ICU discharge. Impaired functioning of such abilities can negatively impact on vocational or avocational tasks leading to significant disruption in life. In spite of this, cognitive recovery does occur, the majority of which happen in the first 6–12 months.

Validated screening tools for ICU delirium:

- CAM-ICU (Confusion Assessment Method for the ICU)
- ICDSC (Intensive Care Delirium Screening Checklist)

Validated screening tools for post-ICU cognitive impairment

- MoCA (Montreal Cognitive Assessment)
- MMSE (Mini-mental State Examination)

3. Mental health issues associated with PICS

- Depression
- Anxiety
- Post-traumatic stress disorder (PTSD)
- Acute stress disorder
- Sexual dysfunction
- Substance use/abuse
- Sleep disturbances

Risk factors for post-ICU mental disorders: (highest in first 3 months)

- Pre-existing mental disorder
- History of alcohol abuse
- Female gender
- Older age
- Lower education level
- Mechanical ventilation
- Longer duration of ICU stay

Psychiatric morbidity following critical illness is the indicator with the greatest negative impact on quality of life for the patient and family. Psychiatric sequelae in such patients can improve but comparatively, it is the longest persisting outcome of PICS.

4. PICS-F

PICS-F (family) refers to a similar range of mental issues being found in family member/caregivers of post-ICU patients. Up to 30% of family or the caregivers of patients experiencing critical illness undergo stress, depression, anxiety, and complicated grief.

Other mental disorders can include sleep dysfunction, PTSD. Psychological morbidity can last months to years following patient's discharge from ICU, with higher rates if the patient does not ultimately survive.

Risk factors can include:

- Poor communication (between family and medical team)
- Family being the primary decision maker
- Lower educational level
- Previous experience with hospitalisation or death of a family member

5. Other PICS sequelae include:

I. Residual fatigue

II. Post-extubation dysphagia

III. Chronic pain

Prevention/mitigation of PICS in the ICU

The **"ABCDEF" bundle** is an evidence-based guide for the coordination of medical and rehabilitation multidisciplinary ICU care (intensive care team, rehabilitation team, etc.) within domains of PICS, and directs treatment to prevent long-term cognitive impairment, delirium, and physical decline in the ICU.

Assess, prevent and manage pain

Both spontaneous awakening trials and spontaneous breathing trials

Choice of analgesia and sedation

Delirium — assess, prevent and manage

Early mobility and exercise

Family engagement and empowerment

The multidisciplinary rehabilitation team in the ICU (Figure 1), looks at different facets of function in the critically ill patient, restores functionality, or mitigate losses early in the patient's journey in the ICU. Regular multidisciplinary meetings can serve to set, align, and prioritize goals, and seeking clarifications (particularly with the intensive care team) where necessary. This is pertinent in the ICU, where the patient's condition can rapidly evolve.

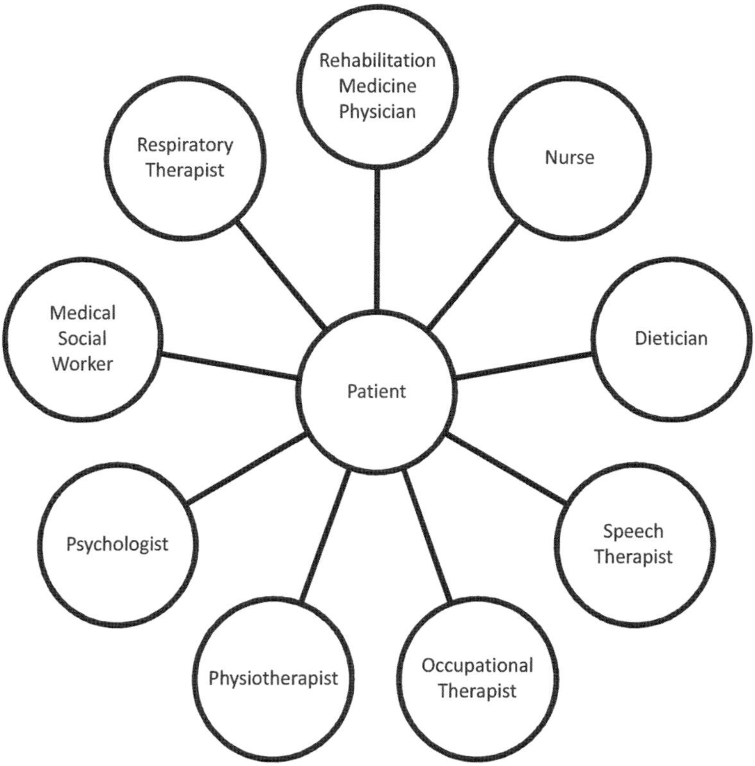

Figure 1. The multidisciplinary ICU rehabilitation team.

1. Early mobility and exercise

Early mobilisation can positively impact on ICUAW and outcome. These include:

- Improved ventilation-free days, functional outcome, discharge-to-home rate, and quality of life
- Reduced ICU and hospital LOS
- Reduced duration of ICU delirium
- Improvements in mood and cognition

Mobilisation involves verticalization and ambulation activities, but can be preceded by in-bed or bedside exercises.

Muscle conditioning activities

- For the awake and cooperative patient, active/active-assisted range of motion and resistance exercises can be started for specific muscle groups. The latter can be achieved with equipment such as weights, resistance bands, or cycle ergometer
- For the sedated patient, passive limb ranging, stretching, and positioning could be attempted. Non-volitional activation of muscles with the use Neuromuscular Electrical Stimulation may be suitable for this group of patients in maintaining muscle bulk, strength, and function

Verticalization and ambulation training

- Verticalization helps to improve orthostatic hypotension secondary to prolonged recumbency, pulmonary mechanics, muscle metabolism and bone health, mood, as well as increasing arousal and awareness. Verticalization also reduces the risk of pressure sores over at-risk pressure points
- Verticalization activities can include assuming a sitting position either in bed, by the bedside or out of the bed (in a chair), propped up in a standing frame, or a tilt-table. These can be precursors to ambulation training if ambulation is not possible. Conventionally, over-ground walking by means of therapist assistance (with or without walking aid) is performed. Body weight supported treadmill training can be explored for such purpose when the early ambulator has insufficient motor control or strength to fully bear weight

An example of inclusion criteria for early ambulation is illustrated in Table 4.

Table 4. Inclusion criteria for early ambulation in the surgical ICU.

Premorbid	• Chair bound/ambulatory
Central nervous system	• GCS (E3-4, M5-6) • Sedation: RASS (Richmond Agitation Sedation Score) +1 to −1 • LL Muscle power ≥ 3/5
Cardiovascular system	• 100 > SBP < 180 • MAP ≥ 65 mmHg • 55 ≥ HR ≤120 • On "low dose" vasoactive drugs • Nor-adrenaline ≤ 0.05 mcg/kg/min • Dobutamine ≤ 3 mcg/kg/min • Dopamine ≤ 3 mcg/kg/min • No new cardiac ischemia or changes to vasopressor dose within the last 24 hours, no new anti-arrhythmic agent

Respiratory	• RR < 30 • Sp02 ≥ 92% • IPAP ≤ 15 • PEEP ≤ 10 cmH20 • Fi02 ≤ 50%
Others	• No surgical contraindications • Pain score ≤ 5/10 • Not pending investigations that might limit mobilisation (e.g. fracture, DVT scan)

Scales for assessment of functional mobility status in the ICU include:

- Functional Status Score for the ICU (FSS-ICU)
- Physical Function in Intensive Care Test (PFIT)
- Chelsea Critical Care Assessment tool (CPAx)

2. Respiratory care intervention and training

ICUAW can also affect respiratory muscles, impacting on ventilatory efforts and secretion management. Although the work of ventilator weaning comes under the purview of the intensive care team, efforts from the rehabilitation team can contribute to weaning success.

Ventilatory assistance

- Breathing techniques can be taught to the cooperative patient and are of particular importance following surgery. Deep inspiration, augmented with a device such as incentive spirometer to provide visual feedback, is a vital factor in reducing/preventing post-operative pulmonary complications. Deep breathing supports the movement of secretions and assists in opening lung spaces that may have become collapsed

- Purse-lip breathing generates a small amount of positive end-expiratory pressure and helps to buttress the small bronchioles, thereby preventing premature airway collapse. With purse-lip breathing, select patients can have relief from breathlessness, reduction in the work of breathing, and improvement in gaseous exchange

- The Positive Expiratory Pressure (PEP) device functions similarly to increase pressure that is transmitted to the airways, creating a back pressure, and stenting the airways during exhalation, thereby preventing premature airway closure and reducing gas trapping.

- Inspiratory muscle training (IMT) has been explored to improve respiratory muscle function and assist in ventilatory efforts. It has been used to improve diaphragmatic muscle strength in patients with ICUAW

Secretion management

- Traditionally, postural drainage, percussion, and vibration (often used in combination) are utilised to facilitate secretion clearance. Strategies such as autogenic drainage, forced expiratory ("huffing") or active cycle of breathing techniques can be taught to the patients to bring up the phlegm. A PEP device can also be trialled to promote mucus clearance
- In patients who are too weak to perform a sufficient cough, manually assisted cough, or use of the mechanical insufflation-exsufflation device can facilitate this task

3. Pain management

Pain is a common problem afflicting patients in ICU. Even though pharmacological management is still the mainstay of treatment, adjunctive pain management strategies can be afforded by the therapists in the form of positioning and physical modalities, as well as cognitive techniques for pain management.

4. Delirium

A large part of the management of ICU delirium focuses on pharmacology management and attenuating modifiable risk factors. (refer "ABCDEF" bundle)

Currently, no single non-pharmacological intervention for prevention/management of delirium in the ICU has been proven to be effective. Despite limited evidence, it would seem rational to recommend multicomponent, non-pharmacological interventions which would seem logical, harmless, and have potential benefit (Table 5).

Table 5. Non-pharmacological management of ICU delirium.

Non-pharmacological management of ICU delirium
• Repeated/daily reality reorientation of patients
• Provisions of cognitively stimulating activities multiple times a day
• Early mobilisation activities
• Timely removal of catheters and physical restraints
• Optimise sensorial inputs (e.g. use of eyeglasses and magnifying lenses, hearing aids, and earwax dis-impaction)

- Early correction of dehydration
- Use of a scheduled pain management protocol
- Non-pharmacological sleep protocol (sleep hygiene)
- Minimisation of unnecessary noise/stimuli
- Realignment of circadian rhythm (e.g. bright light therapy in the daytime)

5. Nutrition

- During critical illness, the body is in a hypercatabolic state, which can manifest clinically as weight loss, sarcopenia, and undernutrition
- Intensive care nutrition guidelines have recommended **hypocaloric nutrition** (not exceeding 70% of energy expenditure at rest) for the first 48 hours of energy expenditure (EE). Caloric delivery can be gradually increased to 80–100% of EE after day 3
- EE should be measured with indirect calorimetry. If predictive equations are used, hypocaloric nutrition (< 70% of EE) is preferred over isocaloric nutrition (> 70% of EE) for the first week in ICU. Proteins should be increased progressively to a rate of 1.2–2.0 g/kg/day (over a week)
- These recommendations are advised for mortality benefits. Thus far, no specific nutritional formulation has been recommended for exercise and physical therapy in the ICU

6. Swallowing

Patients in the ICU are frequently intubated. Post-extubation dysphagia (PED) has been found to be as high as 41% in critically ill adults. And of these patients who were found to have dysphagia, 36% was found to be aspirating silently, and this often requires instrumental assessments for detection. Swallowing impairment may also be evident in patients with tracheostomy tubes.

Mechanisms of PED:

- Mechanical causes (mucosal inflammation, loss of architecture, oropharyngeal disuse muscle atrophy)
- Decreased laryngeal sensation/proprioception, laryngeal injury
- Cognitive disturbances
- Neurological dysfunction
- Prolonged intubation

Risk factors for PED:

- Advanced age
- Pre-existing neurological conditions
- Presence of tracheostomy
- Nasogastric tube placement
- Low GCS scores

Management includes:

- A swallow screening evaluation to determine the need for further instrumental assessment. Instrumental assessments can include investigations such as the videofluoroscopic swallow study or fibreoptic endoscopic evaluation of swallowing — which allows real-time imaging of the different stages of swallowing
- Dietary modification and postural changes/compensatory manoeuvres.
- Direct therapies in oromotor control, such as therapeutic exercises and neuromuscular stimulations are potentially effective treatment modalities that can be considered as well

7. Communication

- Continued dependence on mechanical ventilatory support may result in a situation where the patient is awake, cooperative, and attempting to communicate but unable to do so effectively. This can result in frustration and anxiety, which in turn negatively impact care
- Intubated patients can benefit from communication strategies such as utilisation of AAC (augmentative and alternative communication). AAC can be unaided or aided. Unaided modes of communication can include non-spoken means of communication such as gestures and facial expressions. Aided modes of communication make use of external support. This can be no/low tech such as communication boards with symbols (e.g. pictures, photographs, printed words) or high tech (e.g. computers, handheld devices, tablet devices)
- In a patients with a tracheostomy tube, the use of a speaking valve, leak speech technique, or above-cuff vocalization should be explored as options to enhance communication

8. Mood management

- Pharmacotherapy and psychotherapy are the mainstay of treatment for psychological dysfunction in the ICU. Even then, psychotherapy or counselling is not yet widely used in ICU
- Although not of proven efficacy, various interventions to promote sleep in the ICU (e.g. relaxation techniques, daytime wakefulness, maintenance of a quiet restful environment) have been advocated to promote psychological well-being in the ICU
- Memory gaps are frequently experienced by ICU survivors, and these may be associated with psychiatric disorders. ICU diaries provide a day-to-day record of a patient's admission to the ICU till discharge. They are filled by both ICU staff and families in an attempt to reduce these "memory gaps". ICU diaries possibly can reduce the risk of some ICU-related mental disorders (e.g. depression) and improve quality of life. At this time, its use in mitigating ICU-related post-traumatic stress disorder and PICS-F is not established

Post-ICU rehabilitation

Following ICU discharge, it will be important to evaluate the post-acute impairments. These could be consequent to the disease process and/or part of PICS. Functional evaluation has to be multi-faceted (psychological, cognitive, and physical domains), and would involve assessments by the multidisciplinary rehabilitation team. Rehabilitative interventions, started in ICU, will be continued and likely intensified, with improvements in the patient's condition.

As alluded to in previous sections, despite ICU interventions, many of the multi-domain impairments would persist beyond ICU stay. Some symptoms may linger on for years following ICU discharge, necessitating prolonged continuation of rehabilitation in the community. Regarding physical rehabilitation, outpatient programs vary and can include patient directed exercises, in-home therapist sessions, outpatient clinic sessions, and telerehabilitation.

In some centres, dedicated post-ICU clinics (team-based) are set up to follow up patient who were on mechanical ventilation. Potentially, these clinics would be helpful in detecting, reviewing, and treating post-ICU impairments in ICU survivors.

As awareness of PICS grows, ICU survivorship should be viewed in the same lens as other survivorship programs. The focus needs to be placed on long-term health management and transition of the ICU survivor (from the acute care environment) to the community.

Recommended reading

- Colbenson GA, Johnson A *et al.* Post-intensive care syndrome: impact, prevention, and management. *Breathe (Sheff).* 2019;15(2):98–101.
- Hodgson CL, Stiller K. *et al.* Expert consensus and recommendations on safety criteria for active mobilization of mechanically ventilated critically ill adults. *Crit Care.* 2014;18(6):658.
- Marra A, Ely EW *et al.* The ABCDEF bundle in critical care. *Crit Care Clin.* 2017;33(2):225–243.
- Vanhorebeek I, Latronico N *et al.* ICU-acquired weakness. *Intensive Care Med.* 2020;46(4):637–653.

11

Dysphagia Rehabilitation

TAN Ping Ping, SEE Mei Ting Valerie

Normal physiology of swallowing

In general, there are 3 stages of swallowing:

- **Oral stage**
  Food is chewed into a bolus and pushed to the back of the mouth by the tongue to trigger a swallow
- **Pharyngeal stage**
  The bolus is propelled past the upper oesophageal sphincter into the oesophagus. During this phase, the airway is closed to prevent aspiration of food
- **Oesophageal stage**
  This stage begins when food enters the oesophagus and ends when it passes the lower oesophageal sphincter into the stomach

Dysphagia

Dysphagia is a swallowing disorder, and impairments can occur at any of the stages listed above.

Common causes of dysphagia

- Neurological conditions (e.g. stroke, head injury, Parkinson's disease, motor neurone disease, advanced stages of dementia)
- Complication of surgery from the head and neck region
- Side-effects from radiotherapy
- Respiratory problems (e.g. *chronic obstructive pulmonary diseases* with altered breathing-swallowing patterns may adversely affect airway protection and increase the risk of aspiration)

- Medical conditions that weaken the swallowing system (e.g. achalasia, systemic sclerosis, gastro-esophageal reflux, aero-digestive tract malignancies, etc.)

Symptoms of dysphagia

- Difficulty in swallowing saliva or drooling
- Presence of residue of food/fluid in the mouth after swallowing
- Chewing/sucking difficulties
- Throat-clearing, choking or coughing during or after swallowing
- Recurrent chest infection or fever
- Unintended/unexplained weight loss

Dysphagia in association with cognitive impairments

Swallowing mechanics may be preserved, but safety of swallowing is compromised by:

- Poor visual attention
- Diminished executive functions
- Neglect
- Behavioural issues

Assessment of dysphagia

Examination by the physician before swallowing assessment by the speech therapist include screening for attention span, a brief cognition and language screen, a voice quality screen, pulse oximetry, and respiratory (rate and quality) assessment. A general oral cavity examination including dentition integrity, oro-motor examination (jaw, buccal, lingual, palatal) may be appropriate too.

The Speech Therapist would first perform a clinical evaluation of swallowing. The clinical evaluation include obtaining medical history, case history, a physical examination of the swallowing musculature, and observations of swallowing with test swallows.

When deemed necessary, the speech therapist may request for objective imaging evaluation.

In these objective imaging evaluation, diet (food) and liquid bolus will be presented in various consistencies and modalities. Compensatory strategies may be applied.

The two main imaging assessment are

- Videofluroscopy (VFS) or Modified Barium Swallow Study (MBSS)
  - Advantages:
    - √ Comprehensive evaluation of both oral and pharyngeal phases of swallowing
  - Disadvantages:
    - √ Exposure to small amounts of radiation
    - √ Food is coated with barium hence taste may be altered
    - √ Test may be difficult to perform for patients who cannot sit or be propped (e.g. spinal instability)
- Flexible endoscopic evaluation of swallowing (FEES)
  - Advantages:
    - √ Allows a direct view of larynx
    - √ Portable, and can be done at the patients' bedside
  - Disadvantages:
    - √ No visualization of the actual swallow because of "whiteout" when swallowed material occludes the endoscope tip
    - √ Discomfort
    - √ Potential complications include vasovagal responses, epistaxis, laryngospasms
    - √ However, published reports of large numbers of patients receiving this procedure have documented that this is a safe procedure with few complications.

The speech therapist will evaluate to determine which assessment is most suitable for the patient.

How is dysphagia managed?

- Modification to the size and consistencies of food and fluids
- Environmental modification: Minimize distractions and managing behaviour

- Use of adaptive cutlery and utensils
    - For example, the use of utensils such as a Provale® cup ensures small amounts of liquids are taken at each time.
- Non-oral feeding/enteral feeds via nasogastric tube (NGT) for those who are unable to swallow. For those who need long-term NGT feeding, percutaneous gastrostomy tube insertion can be considered. The advantages of PEG tube feeding include better comfort and cosmesis
    - Compensatory strategies
        - Mendelsohn Maneuver (hyoid lift): Prepare to swallow normally. As you swallow, feel your thyroid cartilage (laryngeal prominence or Adam's Apple) at its highest point and hold it for 3 seconds. Squeeze the throat muscles tight, relax and then repeat for X number of times. This maneuver increases the extent and duration of laryngeal elevation and enhances cricopharyngeal opening.
        - Supraglottic Swallow and Super-supraglottic swallow: Take a deep breath, hold your breath and swallow. A voluntary cough may be performed post swallow to clear any residue from the vocal cords. Extra effort is needed to hold your breath in the super-supraglottic swallow. Both strategies aim to improve airway protection.
        - Effortful Swallow: Swallow hard while pushing your tongue against your hard palate with great effort. The aim is to improve base of tongue retraction, increase orolingual pressure and pressure in the upper pharynx.
        - Oro motor (lip or lingual) exercises
        - Shaker Exercise: Lift your head to look at your toes in a successive or sustained manner while lying flat. This exercise aims to strengthen suprahyoid muscles and increase opening of the upper oesophageal sphincter.
        - Thermal/tactile stimulation of Oropharynx: This is usually through cold stimuli. This helps increase the sensitivity of the oral cavity and may trigger a faster swallowing reflex.
        - Masako maneuver: (Tongue holding exercise) — Stick out your tongue, hold it between your teeth while swallowing with your tongue maintained in this position. The aim is to improve contact between the base of tongue and posterior pharyngeal wall.
- Exercises and compensatory strategies can be used in conjunction with devices such as

- Surface electromyography (sEMG) for biofeedback, often over the submental region.
- Iowa Oral Performance Instrument (IOPI) which provides visual feedback in the training of tongue or lip strength.
- VitalStim® Therapy System, which aims to retrain muscles responsible for swallowing using small electrical currents to stimulate the muscles.

Recommended reading

- Daniels SK, Huckabee ML, Gozdzikowska K. Dysphagia following stroke. Plural Publishing (2019).
- Groher ME, Crary MA. Dysphagia: clinical management in adults and children. Elsevier Health Sciences (2015).
- Langmore SE, Pisegna JM. Efficacy of exercises to rehabilitate dysphagia: A critique of the literature. *International journal of speech-language pathology*, 2015;17(3):222–229.

12

Rehabilitation of Language and Communication Disorders

TAN Ping Ping, SEE Mei Ting Valerie

A summary of commonly acquired communication disorders following a neurological event include the following:

1. **Dysarthria** — impairments to subsystems of respiration, articulation, phonation, resonation, and/or prosody resulting in speech difficulties

   Common types of dysarthria include:

   a. ***Flaccid*** dysarthria — characterised by hypernasality of speech and breathiness and, is usually associated with lower motor neuron lesions
   b. ***Spastic*** dysarthria — characterised by strained or harsh voice quality and, is usually associated with upper motor neuron lesions
   c. ***Ataxic*** dysarthria — characterised by scanning pattern of speech, impaired articulation of consonants and vowels, and abnormal voice quality and, is commonly associated with cerebellar lesions

2. **Dysphonia** — a voice impairment

3. **Aphasia** — difficulties in the expression and comprehension of written or spoken words. Speech patterns of different types of aphasia (Table 1).

   Different classifications of aphasia exist other than the Boston classification system.

   Other classification systems can be based on linguistics, cognitive neuropsychology approaches.

   Determination of aphasia type from brain injuries is more complex than once thought.

   Studies are now showing that the processing of speech and language involves many other cortical and subcortical regions.

   Combination of functional MRI (fMRI) and diffusion tensor imaging (DTI) allows identification and mapping of complex, interconnected anatomical and functional pathways. Greater understanding of heterogenicity of speech impairments in patterns of cortical damage among persons may be eagerly anticipated.

Table 1. Types of aphasia.

	Fluency	Comprehension	Repetition	Commonly associated lesions
Global	Poor	Poor	Poor	MCA (middle cerebral artery), multilobes
Transcortical mixed	Poor	Poor	Good	ACA (anterior cerebral artery)/ PCA (posterior cerebral artery), watershed areas
Broca's	Poor	Good	Poor	MCA, frontal
Transcortical motor	Poor	Good	Good	ACA, prefrontal
Wernicke's	Good	Poor	Poor	MCA, temporal
Transcortical sensory	Good	Poor	Good	PCA, parietooccipital
Conduction	Good	Good	Poor	MCA, arcuate fasciculus

Credits: Handbook of Rehabilitation Medicine, Edition 1

4. **Apraxia** — difficulties planning, coordinating, sequencing muscles for Apraxia of speech
5. **Cognitive-communication disorders** — difficulties with communication resulting from underlying cognitive deficits.

Communication disorders often require clinical assessment tools (Table 2).

Table 2. Acquired communication disorders and commonly used assessments.

Acquired communication disorder	Examples of commonly used assessments
Aphasia	- Boston Diagnostic Aphasia Examination (BDAE) - Western Aphasia Battery (WAB) - Locally developed aphasia tools such as Singapore aphasia test
Dysarthria	- Frenchay dysarthria assessment
Cognitive communication disorder	- Scales of Cognitive Ability for Traumatic Brain Injury (SCATBI) - Cognitive Linguistic Quick Test (CLQT) - Functional Assessment of Verbal Reasoning and Executive Strategies (FAVRES)
Apraxia of speech	- Apraxia battery for adults (ABA)

Rehabilitation of acquired language disorders

Through assessment and collaborative goal setting, the speech and language therapist will develop therapy plans to improve ones' language deficits.

Some common therapies include the following:

- **Response elaboration training** (RET)
    - A therapy technique that involves clinician asking for a response and providing cues to expand on their utterance
- **Verb network strengthening treatment** (VNeST)
    - A therapy technique that focuses on verbs and the formulating of sentences with a given verb. It aims to improve word finding difficulties by strengthening the network of words relating to a given verb
- **Semantic feature analysis** (SFA)
    - A therapy technique that focuses on nouns. People with aphasia will have to describe each feature of a word in a systematic manner
- **Communication partner training**
    - The speech therapist will train communication partners in how to best communicate with a person with aphasia
- **Melodic intonation therapy** (MIT)
    - It involves intoning (singing) to improve expressive language in people with aphasia

Speech Therapists may also recommend Alternative and Augmentative Communication (AAC) systems to supplement communication or speech. These options may be suitable when one has markedly reduced speech intelligibility or severe language deficits impacting on one's ability to speak.

Some low-tech AAC options

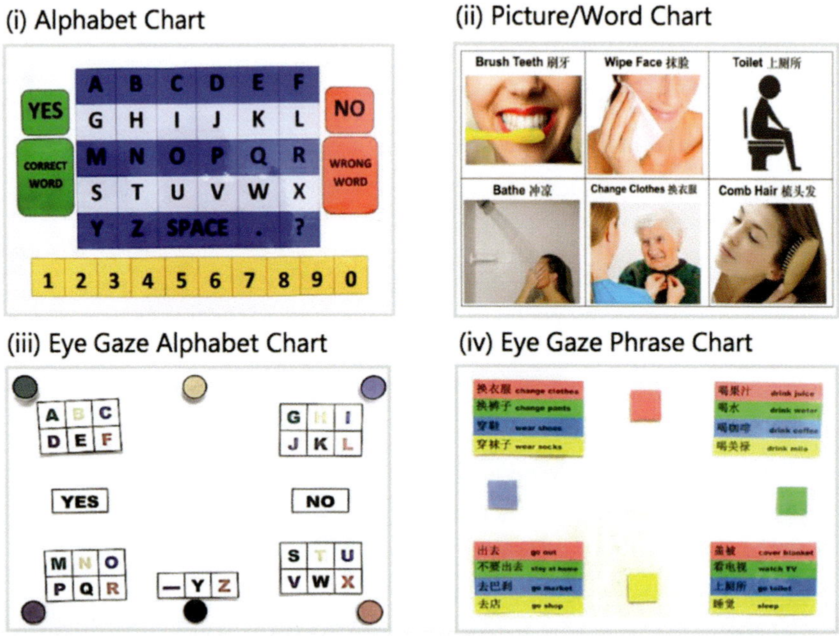

Figure 1. Some low-tech AAC options.
Credits: Tan Tock Seng Speech Therapy Department

Some high-tech AAC options

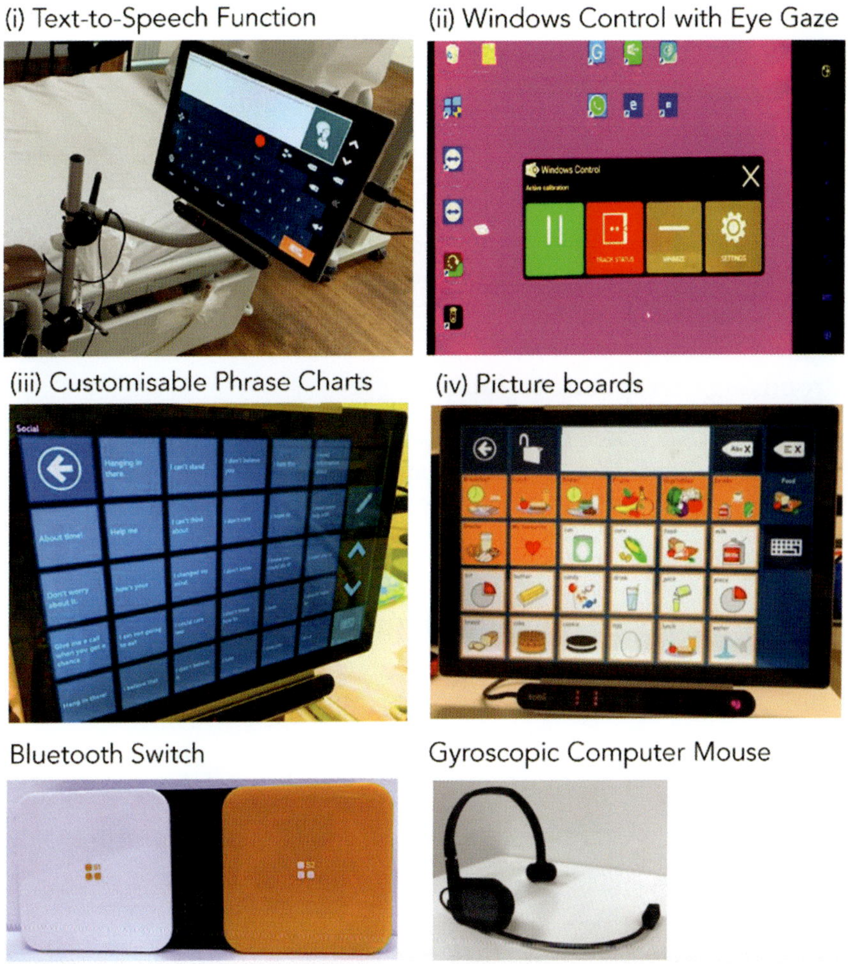
(i) Text-to-Speech Function
(ii) Windows Control with Eye Gaze
Windows Control
(iii) Customisable Phrase Charts
(iv) Picture boards
Bluetooth Switch
Gyroscopic Computer Mouse

Figure 2. Some high-tech options.
Credits: Tan Tock Seng Speech Therapy Department

Telepractice

The use of telepractice for provision of speech therapy has increased exponentially as working remotely and staying at home became a new norm.

Cases suitable for telepractice include:

- Dysphagia assessments for selected patients

- Education and management of dysphagia (e.g. preparation of diet and fluids, monitoring compliance to rehabilitative exercises)
- Dysarthria therapy
- Language therapy
- Cognitive-communication therapy
- Caregiver training in the use of AAC devices in the home setting

Patients can now access therapy services in the comfort of their own homes so long as they have access to appropriate technological devices, basic digital literacy, or a family member to support them if their digital literacy is poor.

Promising therapeutic techniques

Novel therapeutic techniques include neurostimulation techniques using transcranial direct current stimulation (tDCS) and transcranial magnetic stimulation (TMS) to modulate cortical excitability. These are promising therapies to stimulate neuroplasticity and aid language recovery.

General strategies for communication deficits

Consider utilising the P-E-O-P-L-E strategy:

- P –Present 1 idea at a time
- E –Environment: reduce distractions
- O –Observe: use gestures, allow time to respond, observe signs of frustration
- P –Props: use writing/drawing/pictures
- L –Locate trouble in conversation
- E –Encourage when frustrated

Pharmacotherapy and aphasia recovery

Main purpose of pharmacotherapy is to improve and facilitate neuroplasticity.

As language is not a single cognitive function, multiple factors like attention, concentration, memory, and problem solving are involved. This increases the difficulties in the design, interpretation, and application of results of studies to individuals.

Modulating the activities of neurotransmitters with pharmacotherapy that improve language and communication deficits is enticing, but more evidence would be needed to advocate pharmacotherapy.

Most of the positive studies were not designed to show superiority in therapy substitution. Persons should continue to receive multi-/interdisciplinary therapy to promote recovery. Different drugs may be considered for the treatment of aphasia, together with speech therapy (Table 3).

Table 3. Drugs and their possible positive effect in post-stroke aphasia.

Drug	Possible positive effect in post-stroke aphasia
Donepezil - Reversible centrally selective acetylcholinesterase inhibitor - 5–10 mg daily, up to 16 weeks	May help with auditory comprehension, naming, repetition, and oral expression
Memantine - Uncompetitive antagonist of N-methyl-D-aspartate glutamate receptors - 5 mg/daily - May be titrated to max 20 mg/day in weekly increments if tolerating	May help with naming, spontaneous speech, and repetition
Selective serotonin reuptake inhibitors *e.g. fluoxetine, escitalopram*	May help with picture naming, reduce perseveration
Piracetam - A derivative of GABA, γ-amino-butyric acid - May improve the metabolic functions in the ischemic zone - Daily dose of up to 4.8 g/day	May help with auditory comprehension, repetition, spontaneous speech, and written language May help with learning and memory
Dopaminergic agents - *Levodopa* (precursor of dopamine)	May help with repetition and verbal fluency

Recommended reading

- Berthier ML, Green C *et al.* Memantine and constraint induced aphasia therapy in chronic post stroke aphasia. *Ann Neurol.* 2009;65(5):577–585.
- Jorge RE, Acion L *et al.* Escitalopram and enhancement of cognitive recovery following stroke. *Arch Gen Psychiatry*. 2010;67:187–196.
- Seniów J, Litwin M *et al.* New approach to rehabilitation of post-stroke focal cognitive syndrome: effect of levodopa combined with speech and language

therapy on functional recovery from aphasia. *J Neurol Sci.* 2009; 283(1–2):214–218.

- Zhang J, Weu RL *et al.* Piracetam for aphasia in post-stroke patients: a systematic review and meta-analysis of randomized controlled trials. *CNS Drugs.* 2016;30(7):575–587.
- Zhang XY, Shu BH *et al.* The efficacy and safety of pharmacological treatment for post stroke aphasia. *CNS Neurol Disord Drug Targets.* 2018;17(7):509–521.
- Duffy, JR. Motor speech disorders: Substrates, differential diagnosis, and management. Elsevier Health Sciences (2012).
- Chapey, R. Language Intervention Strategies in Aphasia and Related Neurogenic Communication Disorders. 5th Edition, Lippincott Williams & Wilkins, Philadelphia (2008).
- Shrubsole, K, Worrall, L, Power, E, & O'Connor, DA. Recommendations for post-stroke aphasia rehabilitation: an updated systematic review and evaluation of clinical practice guidelines. *Aphasiology*, 2017;31(1):1–24.

13

Practical Approach to Management of Spasticity

TAY Rong Jie Matthew, KONG Keng He

Case study

Mr Tan, a 55 year-old male, had a right middle cerebral artery stroke 3 years ago, which resulted in left spastic hemiplegia. He can walk independently without the use of a walking stick. He now complains of increasing stiffness in his left hand for the past 6 months. Upon further questioning, he states that although he can flex his wrist, he has difficulty extending his wrist. He also has difficulty in extending his elbow when he tries to reach for objects. The patient expresses concern as he uses his left hand to carry and transfer objects, as well as to wear his shirt.

On examination, the patient was unable to extend his left elbow against minimal resistance. His wrist was in a flexed position, and he was unable to actively extend his wrist. Modified Ashworth scale of the left upper limb was graded as follows: elbow flexor (2), elbow extensor (0), wrist flexors (2), wrist extensors (1), finger and thumb flexors (1).

Definition

A commonly cited definition of spasticity by Lance (1980) is a "motor disorder characterised by a velocity-dependent increase in the tonic stretch reflexes (muscle tone) with exaggerated tendon jerks resulting from hyper-excitability of the stretch reflex as one component of the upper motor neuron syndrome."

This definition is useful to distinguish spasticity from other syndromes where resistance to passive joint movement may be present, such as rigidity, dystonia, and contractures.

Notably, a more recent description suggested describing spasticity as "a disordered sensori-motor control resulting from an upper motor neuron lesion, presenting as intermittent or sustained involuntary activation of muscles".

Prevalence and common causes of spasticity

Spasticity can be seen following an insult to the central nervous system, and these conditions include stroke, traumatic brain injury, spinal cord lesions (e.g. multiple sclerosis, suprasacral spinal cord injury), and cerebral palsy.

Spasticity normally develops over a period of time after an upper motor neuron lesion, and although the exact mechanisms have yet to be fully elucidated, it is likely due to reduction in spinal inhibitory mechanisms and changes in the mechanical properties of muscles secondary to paresis.

Estimates of the prevalence of spasticity varies, due to differences in clinical measurements of spasticity. It occurs in 65–93% of patients with spinal cord injury, approximately 75% of patients with severe traumatic brain injury, approximately 1/3 of patients with stroke and around 85% of patients with multiple sclerosis.

Associated signs

Spasticity is only one of the many consequences of the upper motor neuron syndrome. The upper motor neuron syndrome consists of both positive and negative signs.

Positive signs include:

- Exaggerated tendon reflexes
- Enhanced primitive reflexes
- Spastic co-contraction: this refers to inappropriate simultaneous co-contraction of both agonist and antagonist muscles. For example, elbow extension in a stroke patient may appear weaker than it actually is because of co-contraction of the elbow flexors
- Spastic dystonia: this refers to an involuntary posture that may occur at rest or interfere with both passive and active voluntary movements
- Associated reaction: this refers to involuntary movement of the affected body part when the unaffected body part is moved. An example is involuntary elbow flexion in stroke patients as they attempt to stand or walk
- Spasms: these could be extensor, flexor, or adductor spasms
- Clonus: this refers to involuntary, rhythmic, muscular contractions and relaxations due to a self-re-excitation of the hyperactive stretch reflexes in the affected muscle. An example is ankle clonus

Negative signs include:

- Muscle weakness
- Loss of selective motor control with slowness of movements and decreased dexterity
- Fatigue due to greater effort expended in performing a motor task

Common patterns

There are common patterns of spasticity and spastic muscle overactivity that are observed across different patient populations (see Table 1). These patterns can help the clinical team understand the potential complications of spasticity and the upper motor neuron syndrome, and prescribe appropriate therapeutic interventions.

Table 1. Common spasticity patterns.

Most common patterns	Muscles involved	Complications/side effects
Adducted/internally rotated shoulder	Pectoralis major, teres major, latissimus dorsi, subscapularis	• Shoulder pain on ranging • Issues with axillary hygiene • Difficulties in dressing, limitation in reaching forward • Imbalance of gait
Flexed elbow	Biceps brachii, brachialis, brachioradialis	• Difficulties in transfer (no fulcrum), dressing, and reaching • Stretch injury to the ulnar nerve (at the bend of the elbow). The nerve is vulnerable to repeated trauma and can be compressed in the cubital tunnel
Pronated forearm	Pronator teres, pronator quadratus	• Pain on supination • Affects hand function
Flexed wrist	Flexor carpi radialis, flexor carpi ulnaris palmaris longus, long finger flexors	• Compression of the median nerve at wrist with carpal tunnel syndrome • Weakened grip strength
Clenched fist	Flexor digitorum superficialis, flexor digitorum profundus	• Issues with hand hygiene • Difficulties with wearing of hand splints. Limitation of grasping, manipulation, and release of objects
Thumb-in-palm deformity	• Flexor pollicis longus and brevis • Adductor pollicis, first dorsal interosseous	• Difficulty to execute grasp patterns (three-jaw chuck, lateral grasp and tip pinch)

Flexed hip	Iliopsoas and rectus femoris	• Interferes with positioning in chair • Walking with a crouched gait pattern and compensatory knee flexion to maintain balance (leading to fatigability)
Adducted thigh	Adductor longus, magnus and brevis, pectineus, gracilis	• Scissoring thighs interfere with perineal care, sexual intimacy, sitting, transfers, standing, and walking • Difficulties with limb clearance and advancement during swing phase of gait
Stiff knee	Rectus femoris, vastus intermedius, medialis and lateralis	• Interferes with positioning in chair • Gait deviation with the knee remaining extended through the gait cycle • Functional lengthening of the leg during the gait with dragging of the toe and risk to trip and fall
Flexed knee	Medial and lateral hamstrings	• Compensation of ipsilateral hip flexion during stance phase with flexed knee and contralateral hip and knee flexion (crouch gait pattern) • Difficulties with transfers and wheelchair positioning • Limitation of limb advancement due to the lack of knee extension during terminal swing (short step length)
Equinovarus foot	• Medial and lateral gastrocnemius • Soleus • Tibialis posterior and sometimes, tibialis anterior • Flexor digitorum longus and flexor hallucis longus	• Difficulties with shoe wear • Skin breakdown on lateral border of foot • Pain upon weight bearing over the lateral border of the foot • Limitation of heel strike during initial and contact phase of gait • Limitation of dorsiflexion during stance phase with impaired forward tibia advancement, promoting knee hyperextension • Limitation of dorsiflexion during swing phase with impaired ground clearance

Common assessment measures

There are a range of spasticity assessment measures, which can be useful to measure the impact of spasticity and the outcome of treatment. The following are some of the common clinical methods for assessment of spasticity.

Measures of impairments

Modified Ashworth Scale (MAS)

MAS is useful in clinical practice due to its ease and speed of use and is widely used in research. As it measures resistance to passive movement of the joint, it does not clearly differentiate between neurogenic and mechanical causes of hypertonia.

MAS is defined as follows:

- 0 No increase in muscle tone
- 1 Slight increase in muscle tone, manifested by a catch and release or by minimal resistance at end range of motion, when the affected part is moved in flexion or extension
- 1+ Slight increase in muscle tone, manifested by a catch, followed by minimal resistance throughout the remainder (less than half) of range of motion
- 2 More marked increase in muscle tone through most of the range of motion, but the affected part is easily moved
- 3 Considerable increase in muscle tone, passive movement is difficult
- 4 Affected part is rigid in flexion or extension

Modified Tardieu scale

This scale quantifies spasticity by assessing the response of muscle to passive movements at slow and fast velocities. Quantitative joint angle measures are taken at 3 speeds of passive movements: V1 (as slow as possible), to V2 (limb falling under the force of gravity), or V3 (as fast as possible). The corresponding angle is then measured via a standard goniometer for V1 (R1 angle) and V2 or V3 (R2 angle).

The response of muscle to stretch is graded as:

- 0 No resistance throughout the course of passive movement
- 1 Slight resistance through the course of passive movement with no clear "catch" at a precise angle

- 2 Clear catch at a precise angle, interrupting the passive movement, followed by release
- 3 Fatiguable clonus (<10 s when maintaining the pressure) appearing at a precise angle
- 4 Unfatiguable clonus (>10 s when maintaining the pressure) at a precise angle
- 5 Joint immovable

The difference between R1 and R2 is taken as the measure of the dynamic component of spasticity. Hence, a large difference between R1 and R2 suggests that that is a significant dynamic component. The Tardieu scale may be more sensitive in distinguishing spasticity from contractures compared to the MAS.

Range of motion

Passive and active joint range of motion can be measured. Improvement in range of motion can improve splint tolerance and prevent contractures.

Pain

Several measures are available (e.g. numerical pain rating scale).

Spasms

These include the Penn Spasm Frequency Scale and Spasm Frequency Scale.

Measures of activity

1. Passive function: task performed by a carer or by the patient using unaffected limbs
2. Active function: task performed by the patient
3. Mobility (e.g. 10 meter walking test)

Measure of participation — goal attainment scale (GAS)

Patients set their own goals of spasticity treatment in conjunction with the treating healthcare team, before starting treatment. Results of intervention are scored from −2 to +2 as shown in Table 2 below;

Table 2. Results of intervention.

0	Outcome as expected
+1 to +2	Outcome better than expected
−1 to −2	Outcome worse than expected

This is then transformed into a numeric score that allows for analysing group performance. An overall GAS can be calculated when there are several goals, with individual goals weighted by importance and difficulty. It is criterion-referenced rather than norm-referenced, making it responsive to minimally clinically significant changes.

Approach to spasticity

Is spasticity symptomatic?

Define the problem that is affecting the patient. Is it causing pain or affecting passive and/or active function? Input from the patient's carers and managing healthcare team is useful.

Some examples include:

- Relief of pain and discomfort
- Passive function
  - Reduction in burden of care
  - Improvement of hygiene in areas such as the palm, axilla, and groin
- Active function
  - Improve forward reach of the upper limb
- Mobility: Improvement of posture, facilitation of sitting, standing, and walking
- Improvement in body image and self esteem
- Avoiding complications like contractures, pressure ulcers

Not all spasticity has to be treated. Spasticity can confer certain benefits. Knee extensor spasticity allows the patient with weak knee extensors to perform transfers, stand, and walk. Diagnostic nerve blocks can be considered to determine the potential benefits of longer lasting interventions such as chemodenervation or surgery.

Are there aggravating factors that need to be addressed?

Spasticity can be aggravated by certain conditions and noxious stimuli, and these must be ruled out/treated before further adjustments in spasticity management are considered. These factors are mentioned in Table 3.

Table 3. Aggravating factors for spasticity.

Skin lesions	• Pressure sores • Local skin infection or irritation • Ingrown toe nails
Urinary tract dysfunction	• Infection • Urinary tract stones • Incomplete bladder emptying/retention
Gastro-intestinal dysfunction	• Constipation • Diarrhoea • Overflow incontinence
Central nervous system	• Cerebrovascular disease, further stroke/transient ischemic attack (TIA) • Hydrocephalus • Syrinx development
Systemic illness	• Generalised infection • Deep venous thrombosis • Multiple sclerosis pseudoexacerbation/exacerbation/progression
Drugs	• Rapid withdrawal of anti-spasticity drugs • Use of drugs (e.g. SSRI)
Others	• Stress, pain during menstruation • Fracture

Treatment of spasticity

Accurate pre-intervention assessment and intensive post-rehabilitation therapy are crucial for successful management of the patients with symptomatic spasticity, and this invariably would involve a multidisciplinary team.

Physical therapy

Physical therapy includes:

- Stretching: prolonged, sustained stretching to improve the viscoelastic properties of the muscle-tendon unit and its extensibility. Tilt-table standing can provide a prolonged stretch of the ankle plantarflexors
- Casting: a stretching method that immobilises the limb in the stretched position to induce prolonged muscle stretching. Serial casting involves the stepwise application of a plaster or fiberglass cast applied around a joint. The repeated application of casts with the joint being stretched further with each application leads to an improved range of motion, increased function, and/or decreased pain. However, the risk of skin breakdown and neurovascular compromise needs to be considered
- Proper positioning and seating (e.g. in wheelchair) to limit exacerbation of spasticity
- Muscle strengthening and re-education

Physical modalities

Various physical modalities have been used to reduce spasticity, including electrical stimulation (of the antagonist muscles), cold and heat therapy. There is lack of good evidence on the efficacy of these modalities, and even if they are effective, the effects are usually short-lived. More recently, small studies have shown that extracorporeal shock wave therapy is safe and effective in reducing spasticity. Larger studies are needed before this can be considered as standard care.

Orthotic splints

Resting upper and lower limb splints are frequently used to reduce or prevent worsening of spasticity. Donning and doffing as well as skin breakdown are issues to be considered before prescribing splints.

Pharmacological treatment

Medications are generally considered for patients with generalised spasticity (see Table 4). Those with centrally acting side effects, especially the benzodiazepines, ideally should be avoided in stroke and brain injury, as they can cause sedation and cognitive impairments.

Table 4. Pharmacological treatment of spasticity.

Drug	Dose	Administration	Mechanism of action	Side-effects
Benzo diazepines (e.g. diazepam)	5–20 mg TDS	Oral	Increases the affinity of GABA for the GABA-A receptor complex leading to an increase in presynaptic inhibition and reduction of synaptic reflexes	Sedation, weakness, hypotension, confusion, depression and ataxia, risk of addiction with prolonged use
Clonazepam	0.5–1.0 mg OD	Oral	Same as diazepam	Same as diazepam
Gabapentin	600 mg to 1800 mg daily	Oral	Structurally similar to the GABA; acts on alpha-2 delta subunit of voltage dependent calcium channels; mechanism in spasticity unknown	Somnolence, nystagmus, ataxia, headache, tremor
Baclofen	5–20 mg TDS QDS	Oral	Centrally acting GABA analogue; binds to GABA-B receptor at the presynaptic terminal and Inhibits muscle stretch reflex	Sedation, dizziness, weakness, fatigue, nausea, lowers seizure threshold
Tizanidine	4–36 mg daily	Oral	Imidazole derivative, with agonist action on alpha-2 adrenergic receptors in central nervous system	Sedation, dizziness, mild hypotension, weakness, hepatotoxicity
Dantrolene	25–100 mg QDS	Oral	Interferes with the release of calcium from the sarcoplasmic reticulum of the muscle	Generalised muscle weakness, mild sedation, dizziness, nausea, hepatotoxicity

Baclofen should be considered as the first line of treatment for most cases of spasticity, before exploring other drug alternatives.

Chemodenervation treatment

Chemodenervation treatment is the recommended treatment for focal spasticity.

Nerve blocks

The selected nerve is injected with a neurolytic agent, either phenol (5–7%) or ethyl alcohol (45–100%), under guidance of a nerve stimulator. Duration of action can be highly variable depending on the concentration and volume and can range from 3–9 months. Side-effects include pain during injection and dysesthesia due to destruction of sensory nerve fibres. Hence it is most useful in predominantly motor nerves. These include the obturator nerve (adductor spasticity aiding personal hygiene and catheter care) and musculocutaneous nerve (elbow flexor spasticity).

Botulinum toxin injection

Botulinum is a neurotoxin which causes neuromuscular blockade by blocking the pre-synaptic release of acetylcholine resulting in muscle paralysis. The toxin is produced by Clostridium botulinum and seven strains of the bacterium have been identified, labelled A–G. Toxin-A (Botox®, Dysport®, and Xeomin®) is the serotype that has been developed into a therapeutic agent and widely applied in clinical practice. Botulinum toxin-B (Neurobloc®) is also available. However, it is less frequently used due to its shorter duration of action. Units and dosing for different brands of botulinum toxin-A are not interchangeable and are therefore specific to the brand.

It is injected intramuscularly, and muscles to be injected are identified either via muscle palpation, electromyography, electrical stimulation, ultrasound, or via a combination of localization methods. Therapeutic effect is seen in 4–7 days, peaks in 12–20 weeks and lasts for 3–4 months. Serious adverse events are uncommon, and include local and distant muscle weakness. Adjunctive treatment such as physical therapy, stretching, and neuromuscular electrical stimulation can be combined with Botulinum toxin injection. Contraindications of Botulinum toxin injection include motor neuron disease, neuromuscular junction diseases, the use of aminoglycoside antibiotics, and pregnant or lactating patients.

Surgical treatment

Intrathecal baclofen pump

Intrathecal baclofen directly acts on GABA-B receptors in the lumbar spinal cord where a high concentration of receptors allows small doses to be used to good effect without systemic side effects. The intrathecal baclofen pump both stores and delivers programmable doses of baclofen through a catheter into the spinal subarachnoid space. As baclofen is delivered directly to the central nervous system, similar therapeutic effects are achieved with a much lower dose (approximately 1%

of the oral dose), improving spasticity control while reducing side effects. It is indicated for carefully selected patients with severe and refractory spasticity who do not respond to other treatment.

Procedure related complications include infection, skin erosions, and cerebrospinal fluid leak and seroma formation around the pump. Abrupt withdrawal of intrathecal baclofen due to pump failure, battery failure, catheter block, or patient non-compliance to treatment can cause a clinical emergency, with features similar to neuroleptic malignant syndrome which includes high fever, confusion, rebound spasticity, and muscle rigidity. An acute overdose can lead to hypotension, bradycardia/tachycardia, flaccid paralysis, somnolence, delirium, respiratory depression, seizures, or cardiac abnormalities.

Neuro-orthopaedic intervention

These include tendon release (tenotomy) or tendon lengthening, tendon transfers, osteotomies and arthrodesis, neurotomies, and selective peripheral neurectomies.

Management of Mr Tan

So what do we do for Mr Tan, the patient presented in our case study? He has left upper limb spasticity affecting the elbow and wrist flexors which is symptomatic. Firstly, one would like to know whether the patient/carer has been taught stretching exercises, and if not, referral to an occupational therapist may be needed. Secondly, one can consider prescribing oral anti-spasticity medications (e.g. baclofen). Side-effects of sedation and weakness should be explained. On the other hand, as the spasticity is focal rather than generalised, one may go ahead and discuss botulinum toxin injection with the patient. Issues of possible need for repeat injection and costs should be discussed.

14
Assistive Devices and Orthotics

ONG Poo Lee, TAN Llewellyn, HONG Yun,
TOH Ee Mui Shirlene, LIM Pang Hung

Assistive device

Definition

> "any item, piece of equipment or product system whether acquired commercially off the shelf, modified, or customised that is used to increase or improve functional capabilities of individuals with disabilities."

Assistive devices can be broadly classified into the different categories: daily living aids, mobility aids, communication aids, sensory aids, orthotics, and prosthetic devices.

For this chapter, we will focus on daily living aids, mobility aids, and orthotics.

Choosing the appropriate assistive device

The key factor in choosing an assistive device is the suitability of the device. Assessment of suitability is best done through a rehabilitation team, which may include a rehabilitation physician, occupational therapist, physiotherapist, prosthetist & orthotist, and/or speech therapist. Team members may vary depending on the user's abilities and needs. Apart from the user, input from family members and caregivers are also critical in choosing the appropriate assistive device. Other factors to consider include efficacy, reliability, safety, simplicity, comfort, and cosmetics. For high tech assistive devices, one needs to further consider issues like cost, battery life, ease of use, and maintenance. As technology evolves, the range and complexity of assistive devices will increase and it is advisable for the rehabilitation team to keep abreast of the latest assistive devices available in the market.

SG Enable provides an enabling guide in choosing the appropriate assistive device for people with disabilities. This information can be accessed via https://techable.enablingvillage.sg/

A. Assistive device for activities of daily living

Table 1 shows examples of assistive devices that are commonly used to aid in performing activities of daily living.

Table 1. Assistive devices commonly used for daily living activities.

Feeding	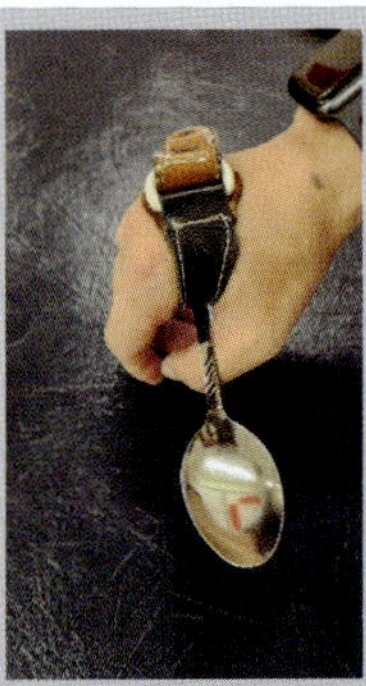 Universal cuff that holds a spoon for self-feeding	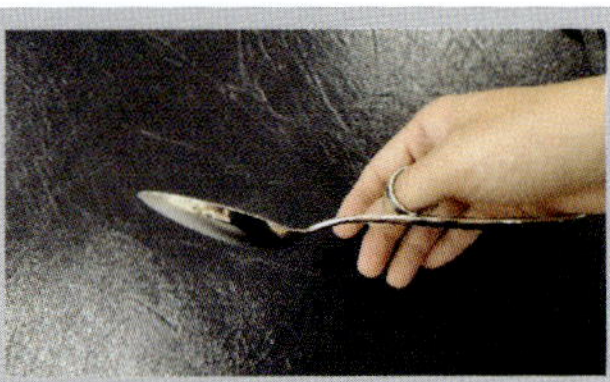 Modified spoon with attached ring for self-feeding
Dressing and grooming	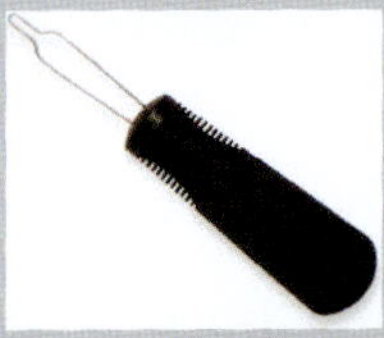 Button hook	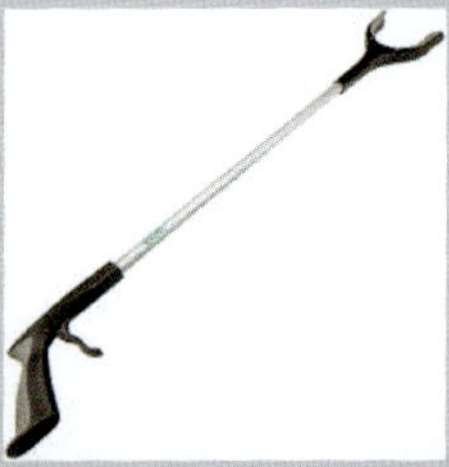 Long handled reacher — helps to pick up items from the floor and cupboards; helps with dressing and reaching and grabbing distant objects

Cooking	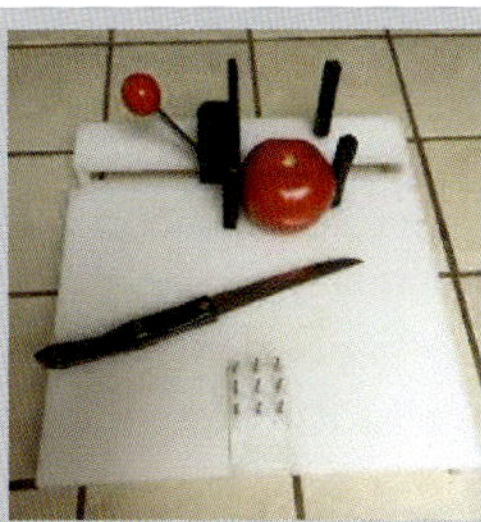 Swedish cutting board — this tool slices, chops, grates and tenderizes with attached stainless-steel spikes that holds food in place, and a vice is available to secure larger items such as mixing bowls; suitable for individuals with mobility or dexterity issues and with only one hand use	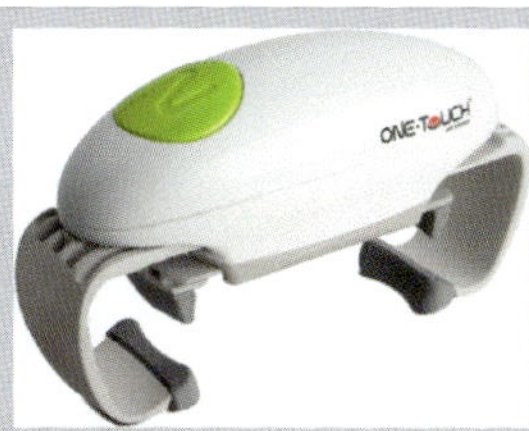 One touch can opener
Writing/ typing	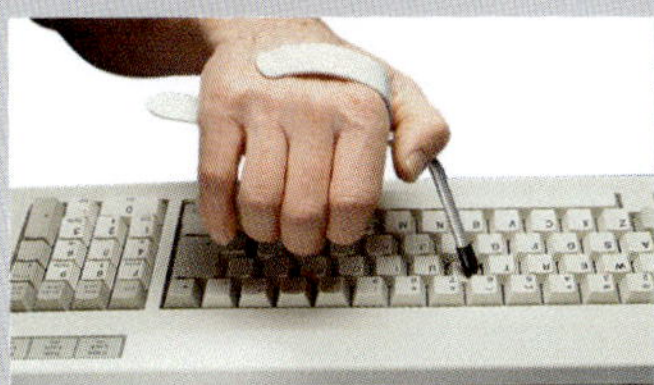 Typing aids	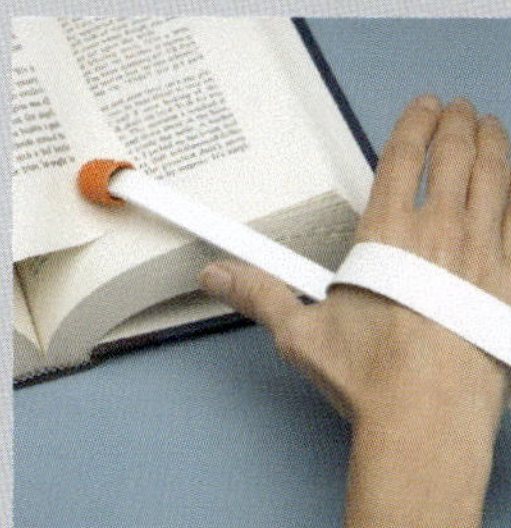 Page turner
Bladder/ bowel	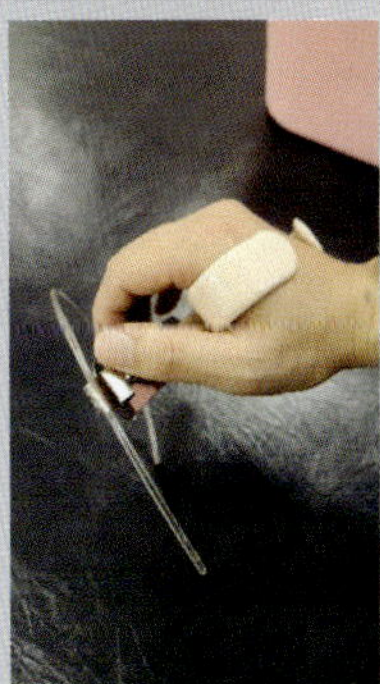 A universal cuff for holding a urinary catheter for self-catheterization	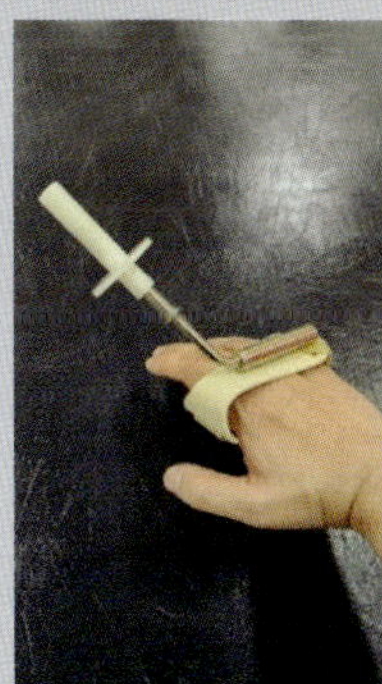 A universal cuff for holding a suppository for self-insertion

B. Assistive device for mobility

Wheelchair

Wheelchair prescription is a process of clinical reasoning. When prescribing a wheelchair, factors to be considered include the person's physical capacity (strength and endurance), physical built, ability to get in and out of wheelchair (transfer ability), purpose of the wheelchair (postural support versus mobility), need for wheelchair maintenance, the person's lifestyle (active versus sedentary), physical environment this person is in (level vs rough terrain), ability to perform pressure relief and re-positioning in wheelchair, mode of transport this person might be taking with this wheelchair, and so on.

1. Lightweight, foldable, detachable wheelchair: these wheelchairs come with detachable armrests and footrests features which allow the wheelchair to be positioned next to the bed/commode/car seat to facilitate transfer (Figure 1). Large rear wheels (22–24 in) are for self-propulsion. Mid rear wheels (16–18 in) are easier for caregivers to manoeuvre. Recommended for individuals who need assistance with transfer
2. Lightweight, foldable, non-detachable wheelchair: these wheelchairs come with fixed armrests and footrests. Recommended for individuals who require supervision or are independent in transfers, but are unable to ambulate for approximately 50 m
3. Push chair/travel chair: these wheelchairs come with non-detachable features and small rear wheels (8–10 in). Recommended for individuals who

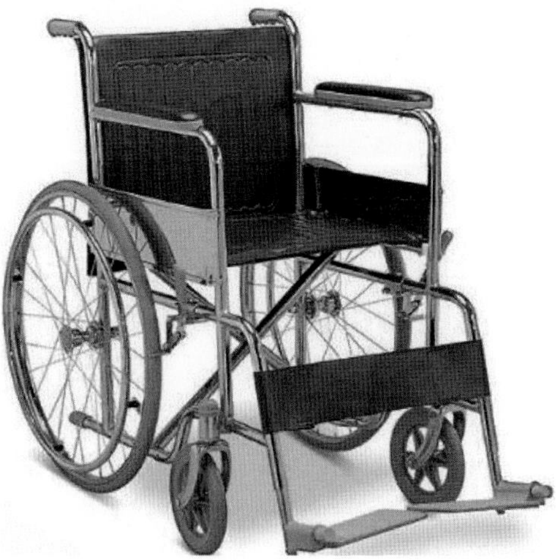

Figure 1. Standard wheelchair.

require supervision or are independent in transfers and are able to ambulate for more than 50 m. Usually used for travelling as it is compact and light (for easy storage)

4. Customised wheelchair: these wheelchairs come with customised features to meet individual needs (e.g. lifestyle and environmental constraints). It is usually used by individuals with no/limited ambulation and are dependent on wheelchairs for their mobility and ADLs
5. Tilt-in-space wheelchair: these wheelchairs come with the power tilt (tilt in-space) feature that allows the whole chair to tilt up to 30 or 60 degrees, while maintaining the hip and knee angles at 90 degrees. (Figure 2)

Tilt-in-space wheelchair

- Promotes proper seating alignment for individuals who cannot maintain pelvic, thoracic, or head position and/or balance against gravity for prolonged periods of time
- Promotes thoracic extension and reduces the risk of respiratory and/or digestive complications
- Provides a change in position without the risk of shear forces
- Reduces the risk of skin breakdown by redistributing pressure from the pelvis to the back

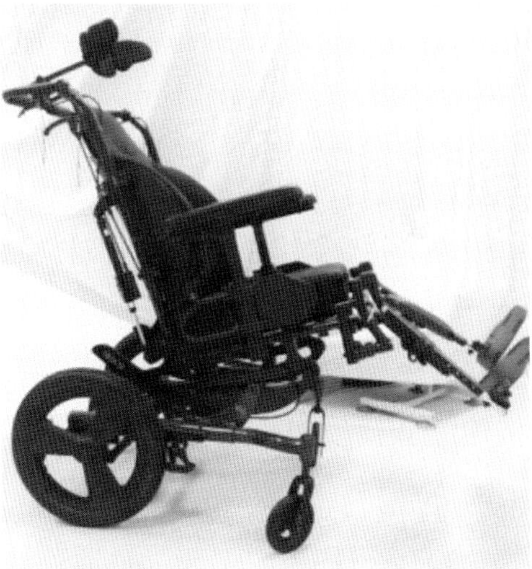

Figure 2. Tilt-in-space wheelchair.

- Provides appropriate position for individual who are at risk of postural hypotension

Walking aids

1. **Axillary crutches (height adjustable)**
   - Purpose
     - Most commonly used for to assist body weight support
     - Not suitable for patients with poor balance
   - Indications
     - Lower limb fractures or joint surgery, requiring partial weight bearing or non-weight bearing of affected leg
     - Lower limb amputation (for pre-prosthetic fitting ambulation or early-stage prosthetic leg gait training)
     - Musculoskeletal injuries to lower limb (e.g. ankle or knee sprain)
   - Advantage
     - Easier to use (than elbow crutches)
     - Preferred by patients with weak upper limb extensor strength
2. **Elbow crutches**
   - Purpose
     - As per axillary crutches
     - Not suitable for patients who have weak upper limb extensor strength
   - Indications
     - As per axillary crutches
   - Advantage
     - Lighter than axillary crutches
     - Easier to manoeuvre at steps and kerbs
     - More trendy designs and colours to choose from
3. **Forearm gutter crutch (Figure 3)**
   - Purpose
     - To be swapped with one side of the axillary or elbow crutches
     - Not suitable for patients with poor balance

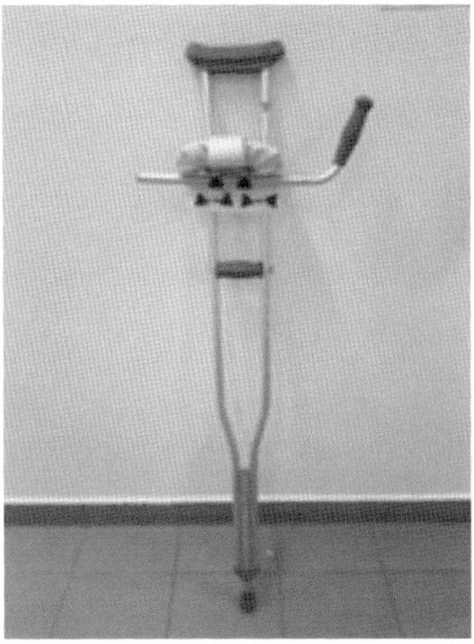

Figure 3. Forearm gutter crutch.

- Indications
  - As per axillary crutches
  - When patient is unable to bear weight through his or her wrist and hand due to injury
- Advantage
  - Avoidance of weight through injured wrist and hand while still using proximal shoulder extensor muscles for assistance in weight bearing

4. Walking Frames (height adjustable)

(i) Regular

- Purpose
  - Commonly used by persons who require help in "body weight support" and/or for stabilising postural control
- Indications
  - Lower limb fractures or joint surgery, requiring partial weight bearing or non-weight bearing of affected leg
  - Lower limb amputation (for pre-prosthetic fitting ambulation or early-stage prosthetic leg gait training)
  - Musculoskeletal injuries to lower limb (e.g. ankle or knee sprain)

- Patients with neurological conditions causing lower limb weakness and/or poor balance
- Frail and weak patients

- Advantage
  - Enhance postural stability due to an expanded base of support over four points

(ii) Rollator walking frame variant (2 wheeled)

- Purpose
  - As per standard walking frame (regular)
  - Set of front wheels allow pushing and gliding of the walking frame over ground hence avoiding actions of lifting and placing of the frame
- Indications
  - As per standard walking frame (regular)
- Advantage
  - For persons who are very weak and/or are unable to lift up the walking frame during walking
  - For persons who have poor balance requiring the expanded base of support at all times when walking

5. Walking stick

(i) Regular (height adjustable)

- Purpose
  - Modestly stabilising patient's postural control
  - Small amount of body weight support is possible
- Indications
  - Mild musculoskeletal injuries to lower limb (e.g. ankle or knee sprain)
  - Mild stroke causing unilateral bodily weakness
  - Need for increased patient's confidence and safety when walking in challenging multi-tasking outdoor environment
- Advantage
  - A light walking aid, easy to carry about

(ii) Umbrella (with rubber tip, fixed height)

- Purpose
  - As per walking stick (regular)

- Indications
  - As per walking stick (regular)
- Advantages
  - Less stigmatising look

(iii) Hiking pole (height adjustable)

- Purpose
  - As per walking stick (regular)
- Indications
  - As per walking stick (regular)
- Advantage
  - Holding onto the vertically oriented handle bar (instead of the usual horizontal handle bar) leads to a more symmetrical postural alignment

6. Quad stick (height adjustable)

- Purpose
  - Useful for both "body weight support" and postural stability assistance, especially in neurological hemiplegic conditions
- Indications
  - Persons with hemiplegic neurological weakness and poor balance
  - Lower limb amputation (gait training with prosthetic leg)
  - Musculoskeletal injuries to lower limb (e.g. ankle or knee sprain)
  - When walking stick is inadequate at stabilising or supporting patient
- Advantage
  - Good stability aid resulting from an expanded unilateral base of support
  - Allows compensation of strength and balance to be derived from the less affected side of the body

7. Platform/forearm support rollator walking frames (height adjustable/ four wheeled) (Figure 4)

- Purpose
  - To assist in heavy leaning body weight support during ambulation training
  - To assist with postural stabilisation during ambulation training

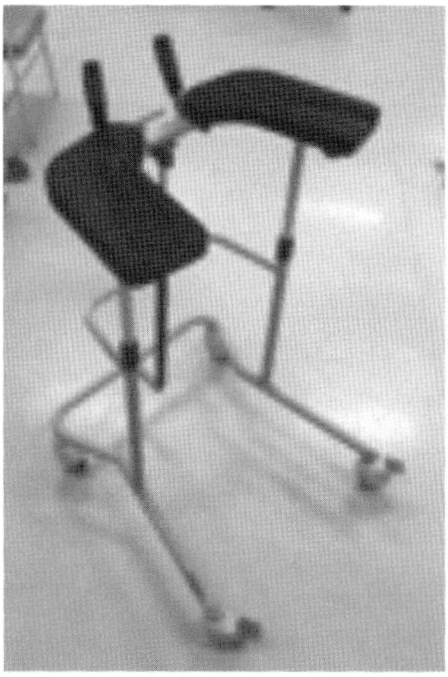

Figure 4. Platform rollator.

- Indications
  - Patients with pronounced weakness and/or poor balance
  - Usually used during early-stage rehabilitation
- Advantage
  - Enhanced stability resulting from an expanded base of support
  - Substantial body weight support through both upper limbs at elbows
  - Reduces effort of walking over level ground, thereby allowing longer duration of practice

8. Walkers (rollators) (Figure 5)

- Purpose
  - A multipurpose walking aid to enhance postural stability and confidence during ambulation
- Indications
  - Older patients with reduced endurance and increased fall risk due to poor balance reaction speed
- Advantage
  - Enhanced stability resulting from an expanded base of support
  - Castor wheels allow for minimal effort in pushing walker (rollator)

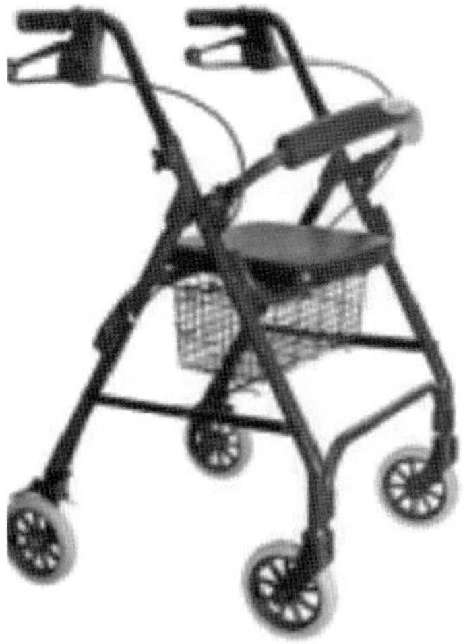

Figure 5. Walker.

- Resting seat is incorporated in walker design
- Designed for in- and outdoor use

Rule of thumb for setting walking aid height

- Walking aid handle height should usually be at the patient's wrist level in the standing position

Coordinated gait pattern when using crutches

- Walking aids that come in a pair (e.g. axillary/elbow crutches, holding 2 quad sticks) will have specific coordinated gait patterns to comply with (e.g. 2-point gait pattern, 3-point gait pattern, and 4-point gait pattern)
- Coordinated and consistent gait pattern will ensure that the appropriate amount of weight bearing for the affected leg is complied with. Patients are also less likely to trip over themselves due to wrong footing

Stair climbing with walking aid

- General rule of thumb for stair climb is to go up the stairs with the "better leg first" and to get down the stairs with the "weaker leg first"
- Walking aid will usually stay with/or follow the weaker leg during the manoeuvre

C. Orthosis

Definition by International Standards Organization of the International Society for Prosthetics and Orthotics,

> "An orthosis is defined as an "externally applied device used to modify the structural and functional characteristics of the neuromuscular and skeletal system"

An orthosis can be temporary or permanent. It can be divided into static, static progressive, or dynamic. The static orthosis has no motion across a joint, while the dynamic orthosis often incorporates springs, pulleys, or strings across a joint to promote function. The static progressive orthosis allows for gradual increase in joint range of motion through use of a non-elastic component that places tension on a stiff joint to hold it at is maximum tolerable length.

Orthoses can be used to achieve the following aim:

- Prevent contractures
- Improve function, mobility or joint movement
- Off-load a joint or body part
- Provide stability for healing
- Correct biomechanical alignment
- Reduce pain

When choosing or fabricating an orthosis, factors to consider include:

- Ease of donning and doffing
- Comfort and cosmesis
- Paying attention to sensitive or tender areas which should be avoided to prevent complications of pain and skin breakdown
- Durability of material
- Cost

Common upper limb orthosis

1. Forearm resting splint

This orthosis is usually used to prevent hand deformities resulting from structural changes associated with neurological conditions, burns, arthritic disease, and injuries. The wrist is commonly positioned in slight extension, metacarpophalangeal and interphalangeal joints in slight flexion and thumb

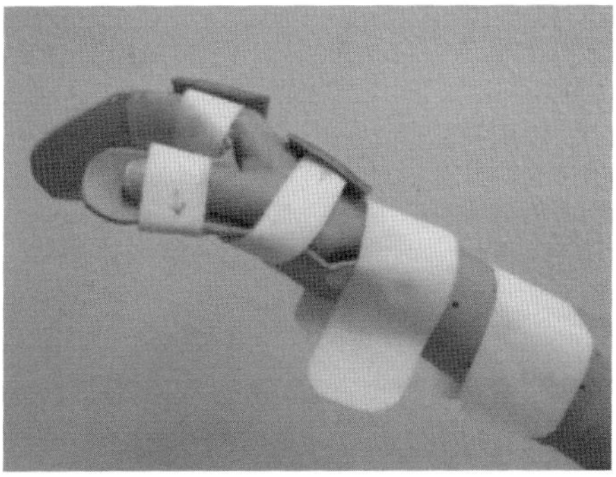

Figure 6. Resting forearm splint.

in opposition (Figure 6). It is used to support normal anatomical hand arches, offering resting comfort.

2. Anti-spasticity hand splint

The wrist is positioned in neutral or slight extension, metacarpophalangeal and interphalangeal joints in slight flexion, and thumb in abduction with 1/3 circumduction. The hand is positioned in this splint to inhibit muscle tone by decreasing the stretch reflex. Splint is fabricated to support hand with moderate spasticity.

3. Wrist cock-up splint/wrist brace

The wrist is positioned in slight extension. This splint immobilises the wrist but allow finger movements. It is used in conditions where a period of immobilisation of the wrist is desired (e.g. acute inflammation of the wrist joint, wrist sprain/ tendonitis, and carpal tunnel syndrome).

4. Tenodesis splint or thumb spica splint

The thumb is positioned in 2/3 circumduction so as to allow opposition of thumb with index finger. Commonly used to provide support for thumb injuries (ligament instability, sprain, or muscle strain), arthritis and thumb sprains. It is also used to stabilise the metacarpophalangeal joints in tenodesis training for individuals with spinal cord injury at C6 level.

Common lower limb orthosis

1. Ankle foot orthoses (AFOs)

AFOs are commonly use in patients with ankle dorsiflexion weakness with resultant 'foot drop'. Common causes include stroke, cerebral palsy, and peripheral neuropathy. The types of AFOs include:

1. Posterior leaf splint (spring) AFO (Figure 7)
   - Usually off the shelf
   - Can also be custom fabricated
2. Supralite AFO (variant of posterior leaf splint)
   - Off the shelf
   - Lightweight and highly flexible
3. Solid AFO (Figure 8)
   - Custom fabricated
4. Hinged AFO
   - Custom fabricated from a solid AFO
5. Anterior support (Toe-Off) AFO
   - Off the shelf with minor customisation possibility
   - Light and strong fibreglass material
6. Ground reaction force AFO
   - Custom fabricated
   - Specialised custom made AFO to assist patients who are weak at the hip/knee extensors resulting in excessive knee flexion in standing and walking posture (usually the problem occurs bilaterally in both limbs)

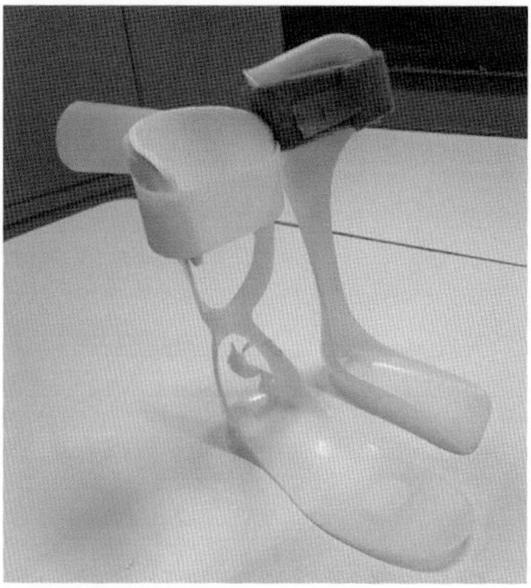

Figure 7. Posterior leaf splint AFO.

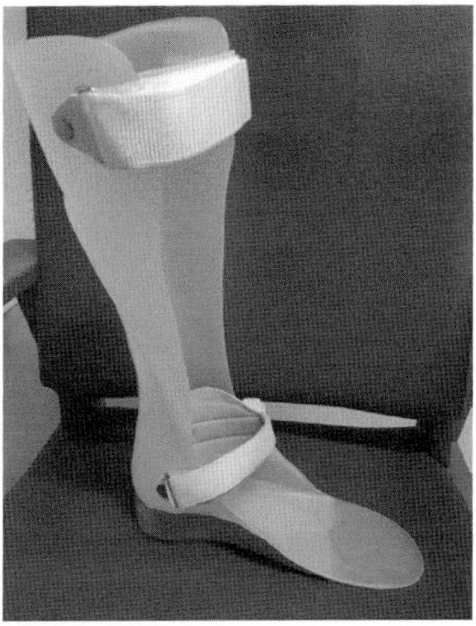

Figure 8. Solid AFO.

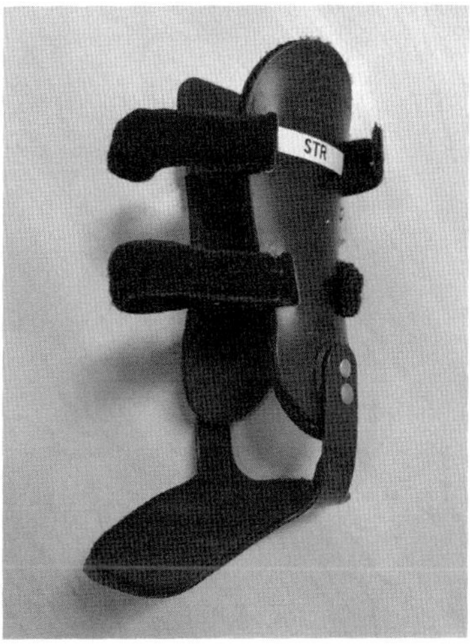

Figure 9. Surestep.

7. Surestep, lateral support AFO
   - Off the shelf (Figure 9)
8. Resting AFO/night splint
   - Usually off the shelf but will need custom fabrication if strong spasticity or severe contracture is present (Figure 10)

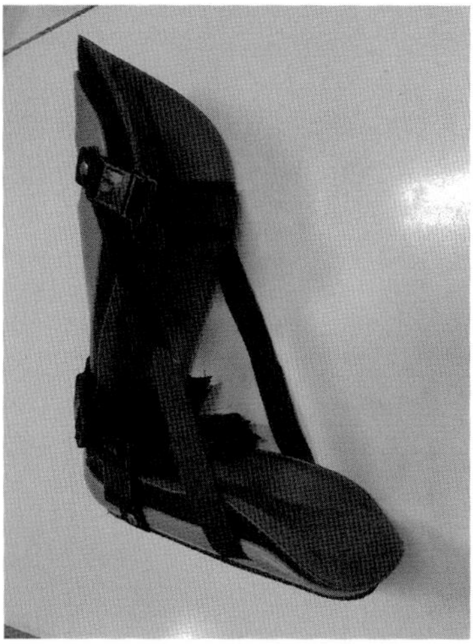

Figure 10. Resting AFO.

Key considerations in addressing AFO requirements

1. **Complexity of joint misalignment encountered during walking**
   - For simple foot drop correction, foot lifting forces provided through an AFO like the posterior leaf splint, may achieve sufficient ground clearance required during "initial swing" phase in gait
   - Complex issues faced during pre-swing in gait cycle may include strong involuntary ankle foot dynamic synergy. This results in twisting action at the forefoot and ankle producing forefoot supination and ankle plantarflexion (equinus foot)
   - Such situation may require custom made solid AFO that wraps around the forefoot and ankle to restrict supination and a strong dorsum strap to restrict plantar flexion
   - In certain cases, a more flexible off the shelf lateral support AFO like the Surestep (fixed) AFO may be sufficient to restrict the equinus tendency
2. **Step pattern**
   - Normal gait efficiency is highly derived from the "rear-foot" and "forefoot" rocker mechanisms. In a gait cycle, these mechanisms occur during:
     - Initial contact (initial stance or "heel strike")
     - Terminal stance ("push-off" or pre-swing)

- All AFOs can allow the rear foot rocker mechanism to take place if the patient has sufficient control and power to generate the forward propulsion momentum, but only AFOs with sufficiently soft and flexible under sole material can allow the forefoot rocker mechanism experience (e.g. the Supralite posterior leaf AFO, or a posterior leaf AFO that has the length of its plastic sole ending just before the ball of the foot)
- The forefoot rocker mechanism is especially important for patients who are progressing in their gait ability, taking larger step lengths, and generating higher forward movement momentum
- Specially designed anterior support AFOs are supposed to enhance patient's effort to engage the forefoot rocker mechanism (e.g. the Toe-Off AFO). Such AFOs do require patients to have a sufficient level of strength and control in their gait in order to generate and benefit from the "energy return" offered by the orthotic device during the push off/ terminal stance phase in gait
- A solid AFO on the other hand will totally prevent the occurrence of forefoot rocker action
- An alternative method to mimic the forefoot rocker action in the solid AFO is to design and incorporate a hinge that allows dorsiflexion > 90 degrees and stops plantar flexion at about 90 degrees

3. **Ease of wearing**
   - Shape and size of the AFO's sole portion should be slim enough to slip into shoes easily

4. **Comfort**
   - The plastic edges of an AFO must not bend into the skin of the foot and calf
   - Padding should cushion the patient's skin against the AFO material (especially at the weight bearing areas). Otherwise socks should be worn before wearing the AFO

5. **Aesthetics**
   - AFOs should not look excessively bulky and cumbersome

2. <u>Knee ankle foot orthoses (KAFO)</u>

KAFO is usually prescribed to improve stability of the knee joint as a result of joint laxity or weakness (Figure 11). It provides stability during the loading response of the gait cycle by preventing excessive knee flexion or during mid-stance to terminal

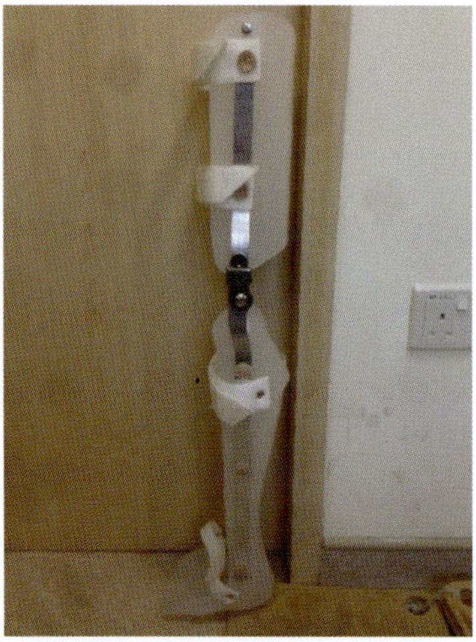

Figure 11. Knee ankle foot orthoses (KAFO).

stance by preventing knee hyperextension. Traditional KAFOs usually maintain full knee extension on ambulation. This leads to hip hiking, circumduction of the limb, or vaulting on the contralateral side in order to advance the limb forward. All of these gait deviations can result in long-term musculoskeletal complications.

3. **Knee orthosis (KO)**

Swedish knee cage

- Use to control minor to correct genu recurvatum caused by ligamentous or capsular laxity (Figure 12)

Ranger knee brace

- Has adjustable knee joints that can be locked to limit knee range of motion control follow surgery or ligamentous injury (Figure 13)

4. **Spinal orthoses**

Spinal orthoses are mainly used for the following purposes:

- Immobilisation and stabilisation of the spine to allow for recovery after spinal injury or post-operatively
- Restricting spinal range of motion for pain relief
- Correction of deformity (e.g. scoliosis or kyphosis)

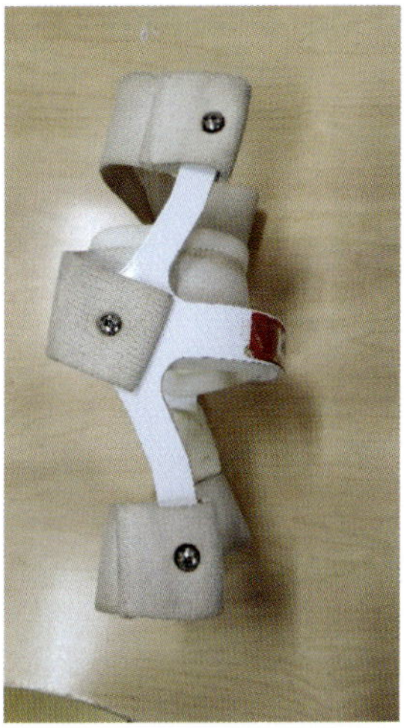

Figure 12. **Swedish knee cage.**

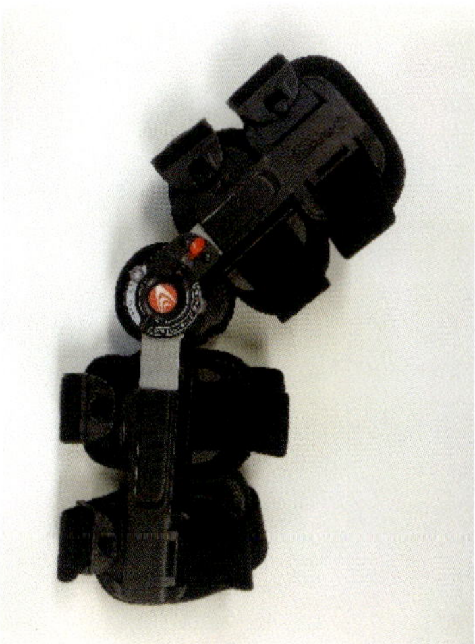

Figure 13. **Ranger knee brace.**

An orthosis that is too tight can cause discomfort (e.g. difficulty in breathing, swallowing, and coughing). A loose orthosis will lose its purpose of immobilisation of the spine.

The fit of the orthosis should be reviewed regularly, in particular, looking for pressure ulcers over areas of bony prominence.

Examples of common spinal orthoses in clinical care are as follows:

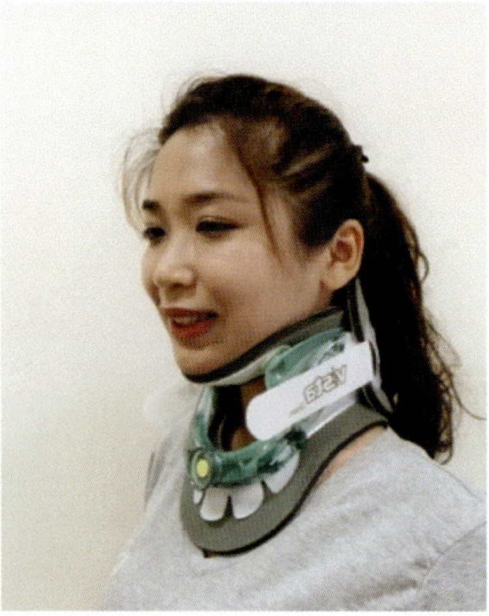

Figure 14. Cervical orthoses (aspen collar).

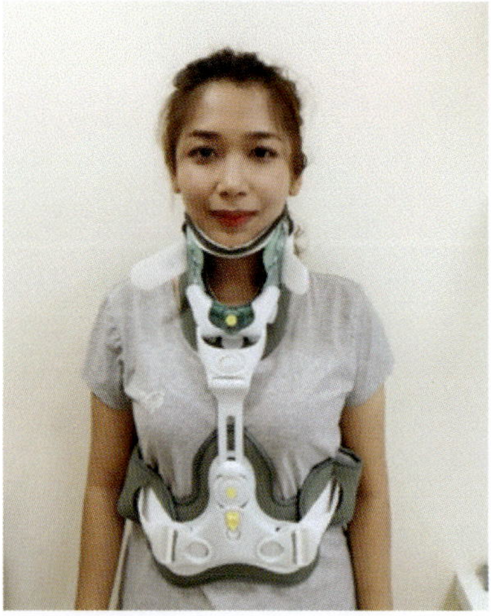

Figure 15. Cervical thoracic orthosis.

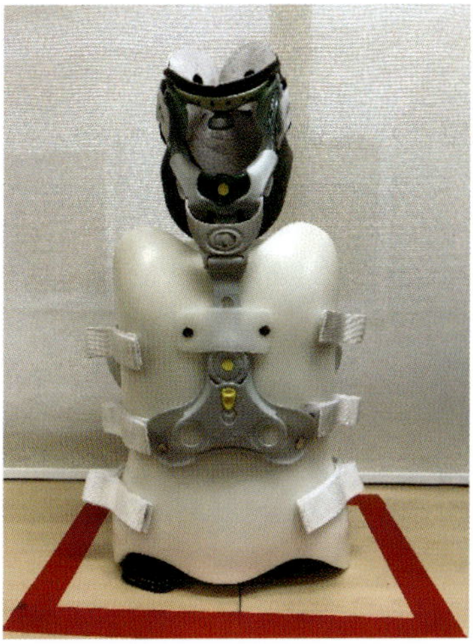

Figure 16. Cervical thoracic lumbar orthosis (CTLSO).

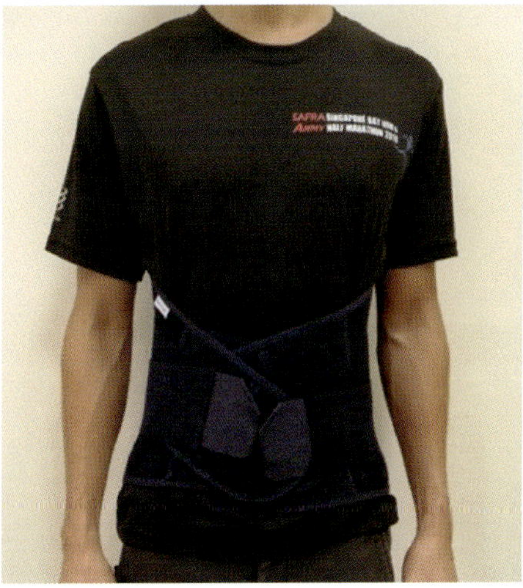

Figure 17. Lumbar corset.

Case illustration

Mr A is a middle-aged man who suffered a spinal cord injury as a result of a motor vehicle accident when he was 24 years old. His neurological level was C6, ASIA A, meaning that he had limited distal upper limb motor power, and absent lower limb motor power. Currently, he's working as an administrative staff and lives with a domestic helper in an apartment. He is generally independent in his ADLs and moves about in a wheelchair. He uses a universal cuff to assist with brushing of his teeth and feeding. He enjoys playing video games and has a 3D printed joystick with adapted grip attached to his gaming unit. Mobility-wise, he is a very active person and enjoys playing tennis. As such, a customised lightweight wheelchair with vinyl coated push rims that allows for better wheelchair propulsion was prescribed.

Mr A's apartment is very much a smart home. He accesses his apartment via a digital lock and remotely controls the air conditioner, lights, motorised window shades, and television via his smartphone. This has greatly enhanced his independence and reduced dependence on his domestic helper, something which would not likely be possible in the past.

15

Clinical Perspectives on Rehabilitation Technology

CHUA Sui Geok Karen, WEE Seng Kwee,
KUAH Christopher, LOH Yong Joo

Introduction

Over the past 3 decades, the advent of technological devices to augment clinical rehabilitation practice has brought great promise and potential.[1] The deployment and adoption of novel restorative rehabilitation technology has also become pervasive due to an increasing evidence base, widespread availability, and lower cost. Robot-aided therapy (RAT) can deliver precise, guided, repetitive, and reproducible movements by 10-fold compared with conventional therapy with high levels of safety and acceptability. RAT can be paired with virtual reality (VR) platforms to motivate and augment user experience. Overall, reduced human effort and fatigue for both patients and therapists make RAT an acceptable and feasible complement to conventional rehabilitation therapies.

In this chapter, we highlight the major types of rehabilitation technologies used in clinical practice for locomotor training, upper limb rehabilitation, including wearable technologies, virtual reality (VR) applications, and brain computer interface, highlighting how technology works, its evidence, clinical applications and practice.

A. Robotics in rehabilitation of locomotor function

Regaining the ability to walk is often regarded as a top priority in patients with various neurological disorders. Manual assistance to facilitate every step of the patient in gait training sessions can be extremely labour-intensive; often, 2 or more therapists are required to support a very dependent patient who is relearning to ambulate. Robotic technology can aid patients to practise up to 1000 steps in 30 minutes of therapy compared to conventional physiotherapy, whereas patients with moderate to severe level of dependence achieve an average 100 steps in 30 minutes of therapy.

In addition to strengthening the trunk and lower limbs, improving coordination, and walking endurance, other non-locomotor benefits of robot-assisted therapy include reduction in spasticity and pain, increased lean body mass and bone density, improved bowel and bladder functions, and improved psychological well-being.

Currently, the most widely used robotic technology include: (i) Treadmill-based robotic gait systems and (ii) Robotic exoskeletons.

(i) Treadmill-based robotic gait training systems

The treadmill-based robotic gait training system, such as the Lokomat® (Hocoma AG, Switzerland) (Figure 1) and ReoAmbulator® (Motorika, New Jersey, USA), uses a body weight support system with safety harness to suspend individuals while their legs are attached to robotic legs that assist with basic walking functions through programmed physiological gait cycles which can be individualised. Virtual reality games built into the system help to engage and motivate patients.

Patients with severe neurological conditions who are maximally dependent, with poor trunk control, will benefit most from the fully supported system to commence weight bearing through the affected extremities, and begin safe, early, and intensive locomotor training that offers an average of 1000 repetitive gait cycles per half an hour of treatment period. Treadmill-based robotics training works best for patients who are unable to walk or need total assistance of 2 persons to walk.

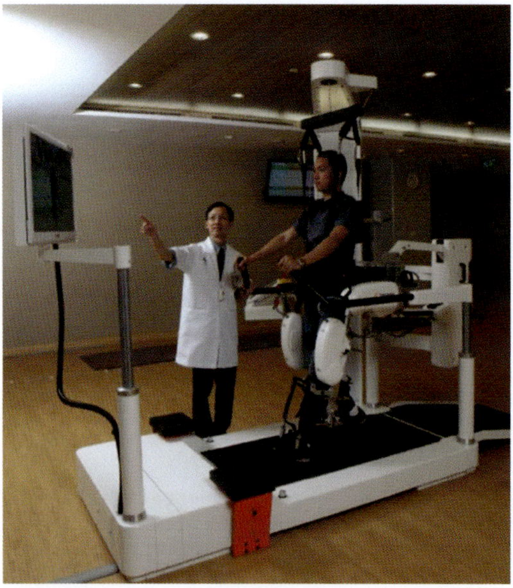

Figure 1. Lokomat (Hocoma AG, Switzerland).

One limitation of this training system is that balance training is under-challenged due to the presence of the body harness (for unweighting) and limb orthoses. Therefore, it is imperative to combine RAT with conventional balance training and overground ambulation to augment the benefits of RAT. Fear of the system, skin abrasions from the trunk and pelvic harness or musculoskeletal injuries (pain, swelling, fractures, superficial contusions) from the harness or boredom during repetitive training are some disadvantages. Fortunately, these are uncommon occurrences.

(ii) Robotic exoskeletons

Wearable robotic exoskeletons are promising new rehabilitation therapies that can provide high-intensity overground gait training. Examples of such exoskeletons include Ekso GT® (Ekso Bionics, Richmond, California, USA) (Figure 2), ReWalk® (ReWalk Robotics (Yokneam Ilit, Israel), Indego® (Ekso Bionics, USA), and Hybrid Assistive Limb® (Cyberdyne Inc, Tsukuba, Japan).

The robotic exoskeleton minimises users' abnormal posture and movement and enable them to experience walking in a normal physiological gait pattern as

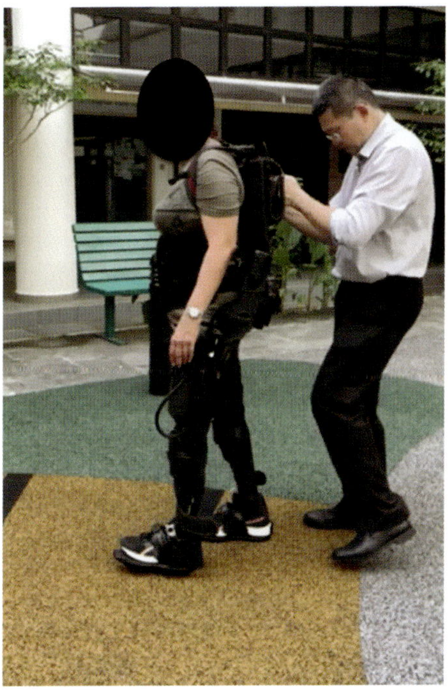

Figure 2. Ekso GT.

part of motor relearning. Due to the nature of intensive gait training, using an exoskeleton has the potential to improve patients' gait pattern, gait efficiency, and cardiovascular fitness. In addition, the trunk muscles, control, and balance may also be activated as a result of sustained upright posture and dynamic weight shifting. In contrast to tethered treadmill-based robotic gait training systems, wearable robotic exoskeletons also enable gait training in varied non-gym settings such as rehabilitation wards, outdoor terrains (gentle slopes, uneven surfaces) or common spaces. This feature provides closer to real-life experiences, making rehabilitation more engaging. In addition, visual spatial and vestibular components are entrained as the user navigates on different environmental surfaces.

Customisation, adaptive control, and progression of various components of gait parameters, including level of assistance from the robot, step height, step length, and swing speed are provided to promote active participation and motor relearning by the user that is reasonably challenging, even for those who are too weak to initiate active weight shifting and swing through of the lower limb during the gait cycle. Certain models of exoskeletons can be used as home-based personal mobility devices with a period of intensive carer and patient dyadic training.

There are limitations in the current robotic exoskeletons; majority of commercial exoskeletons lack self-balancing features which can minimise fall risk although these will increase device weight. Due to high cognitive demands to constantly maintain trunk and balance control, weight shift, and limb activation to swing through, those with severe cognitive or attentional impairments may not be suitable.

In conclusion, with increasing evidence to support RAT to improve trunk control, lower limb strength, coordination, balance, walking ability as well as autonomic function, well-being and quality of life, rehabilitation professionals have available technological tools to augment conventional physiotherapy approaches to optimise mobility outcomes and enhance productivity. Further enhancement to robotic gait training systems will potentially increase the adoption and use in clinics, homes, and community.

B. Robotics for rehabilitation of upper limb functions

Recovery of the arm and hand for functional use remains a key challenge of neurorehabilitation for the enhancement of participation in life roles and quality of life. Conventional upper limb rehabilitation session has been shown to achieve as low as 32 arm movement repetitions per session versus a robotic-based session hitting about 1000 repetitions. Hence, robotic-based training allows for a therapy paradigm of increased training dosage and one that accords with motor learning principles, that can improve daily living activities, arm function and strength post-stroke.

Clinically, robotic training maybe indicated for different intentions such as motor recruitment in the subacute stage versus muscle recruitment for task performance and spasticity management for more stabilised users or those in the chronic stage.

Types of robot design

Upper limb robotic trainers are designed with different functionalities in mind and can be classified according to their technological features and clinical applications. Targeting the arm for reach training may involve shoulder, elbow, and/or wrist movements and those of the hand may include various types of grasping patterns. Training can be in 2 or 3 dimensional planes, and mobilisation include passive, assisted-as-needed or active-based modes.

Non-portable robotic devices tend to be also tethered to a computer workstation incorporating interactive gameplay that can be calibrated to elicit and optimise movement output and to make training fun. Auditory and visual outputs provide encouragement and feedback. Users are also able to keep track of their progress through performance reports and technology-based assessments conducted using the robots when available.

(i) Exoskeleton robot

With multiple rigid frames and device joints axes in line to anatomical ones, large range of movements in 3-dimensional workspace can be trained (Figure 3). Such design can potentially provide better support to reduce compensatory and/or abnormal synergistic patterns. However, they tend to be heavyset and are more complex to operate.

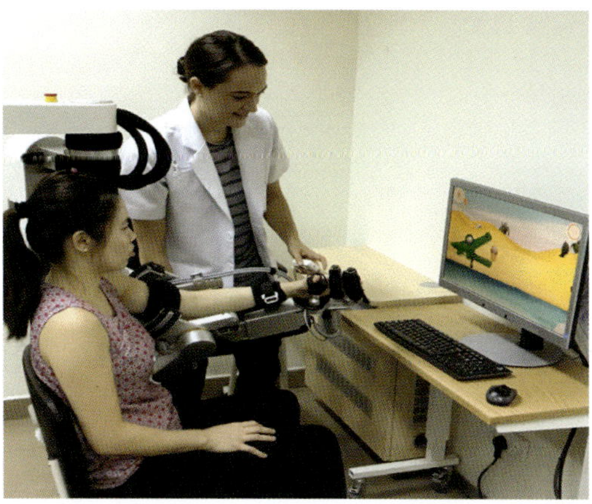

Figure 3. Hocoma ArmeoPower.

(ii) End-effector robot

In such a design, the user's arm or hand interfaced with the robot distally, such as, holding onto a handle for shoulder-elbow training or fingertips attached to the device for hand training (Figure 4 and Figure 5). Similar to the exoskeleton robot, wheelchair users are able to access such systems as they are not meant to be portable while in training use. Although allowing for quick setup for varying arm lengths or hand size and possibly self-operation, reduced support may be needed for very weak arms.

(iii) Soft robotics and exosuit

More recent advances have seen the development of wearable soft robotics. Pneumatic or cable-driven exosuits and glove-based devices consist of soft compliant textiles with minimal rigid elements worn on the arm or hand to

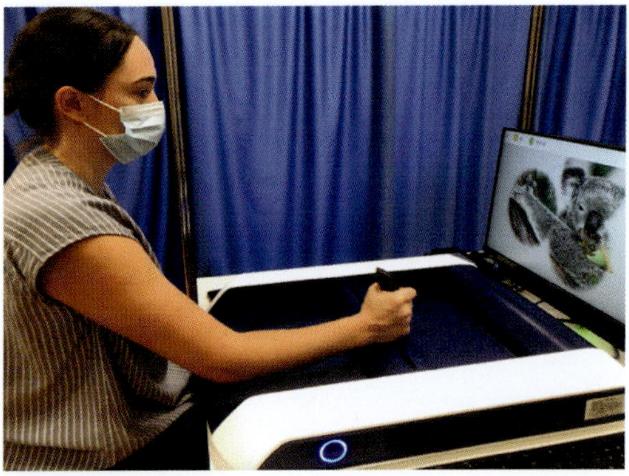

Figure 4. Articares H-MAN.

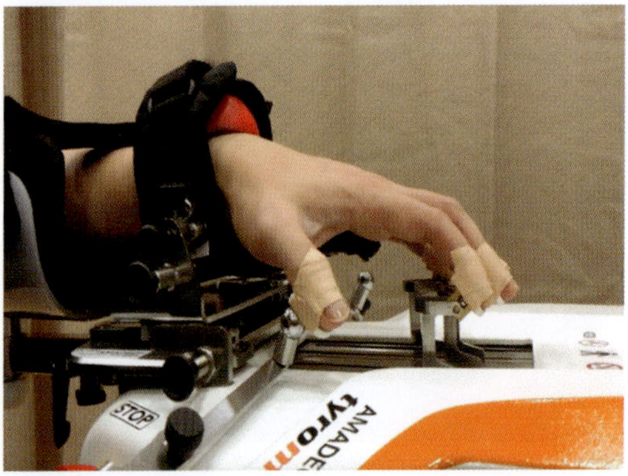

Figure 5. Tyromotion Amadeo.

support participation in activities of daily living. Being lightweight and hence portable, it is potentially beneficial for both rehabilitative and assistive functions, and may reduce user fatigue by reducing muscular activity.

Practice integration and expansion

Key to a successful program is a combinatory approach incorporating evidence and pragmatism. Robotics therapy should be leveraged upon not only for increased engagement and practice, but therapists' work productivity too. It has to be integrated with conventional therapy incorporating individualised goals, involvement of task-oriented and activities of daily living training, and home training program. Support systems to provide efficient technical support, staff upskilling, and program evaluation and refinement are critical to ensure clinical efficiency, relevance, and adoption.

In a push towards hospital-to-home applications, robot trainers have also been incorporated into tele-rehabilitation exercise platforms. Such an approach to decentralise and increase access to high quality care even at home can be facilitated by developing smart, portable, and remote-monitoring enabled devices.

C. Virtual reality rehabilitation

Virtual reality (VR) rehabilitation may be defined as the use of interactive simulations to provide rehabilitation users with opportunities to engage in environments that appear and feel similar to real-world objects and events. It involves the use of advanced human-computer interfaces, allowing users to be immersed in computer-generated environments in a naturalistic fashion.

VR-based technology (VRT) consists of implementing VR using multimedia devices to allow individuals to interact with a VR environment (VRE). While sensory information (visual, auditory, haptic) are transmitted to users, data related to users' actions (motions, gestures, and speech) are also collected to improve the progression of computer games.

Augmented reality (AR) refers to an interactive experience of a real-world environment where the objects that reside in the real world are enhanced by computer-generated perceptual information.

Mixed reality (MR) refers to the merging of real and virtual worlds to produce new environments and visualizations, where physical and digital objects co-exist and interact in real-time).

VR environments can be divided into various degrees of immersion depending on the level of isolation from the physical world; i.e. non-immersive (traditional computer screen or tablet), semi-immersive (large 3D screen), or fully-immersive VREs (360 screens or head-mounted displays). (Table 1)

Table 1. Examples of VR rehabilitation systems.

Immersive VR rehabilitation systems	Non-immersive VR rehabilitation systems
1. Cave Automatic Virtual Environment (CAVE) rehabilitation systems (for research purposes)	1. Commercial Off-the-Shelf Consoles (COTS) • Nintendo Wii • Xbox Kinect
2. Computer Assisted Rehabilitation Environment (CAREN) rehabilitation system: versatile, multi-sensory virtual reality system used for treatment and rehabilitation of human locomotion, or walking, as well as pain, posture, balance spinal stability, and motor control integration	2. Customised VR rehabilitation systems: • Jintronix ® • Neuroathome ® • Silverfit ® • Mindmaze
3. Gait Real-time Analysis Interactive Lab (GRAIL) rehabilitation system: uses all available gait parameters for real-time data collection and visual feedback for effective and motivating gait and balance therapy	3. Mobile digital rehabilitation applications (trial phase)
4. Customised immersive goggles rehabilitation systems: dancing minds	4. VR augmented robotics rehabilitation systems: • Lokomat ® • Armeo ® • HMAN ® • Balance motus

Most are currently available except for mobile apps on trial phase CAVE mostly for research.

Advantages of using VR systems

- Provision of highly intensive and repetitive exercises to maximise motor learning and neuroplasticity to restore function and abilities in those with physical and cognitive impairments
- Integration of physical task into motor activities that require active core or limb movements to control the VR experience, including entrainment of cognitive content to increase motivation and enjoyment
- Allowing an individual to interact in a safe, non-threatening, and realistic environment
- Provision of personalised feedback and prescriptive programmes which can be tailored to patient needs

- Potential for lowered costs of treatment compared with other advanced rehabilitation therapies (e.g. robot-assisted therapies), where it can be used independently by the patient, and it is adaptable for semi-independent home use with or without tele-rehabilitation functions

Potential side effects of VR rehabilitation

(i) Simulator sickness:
A type of motion sickness characterised by discomfort, fatigue, nausea, and disorientation. It arises from the discrepancy between a more vigorous motion perceived by vision and hearing and a weaker motion perceived by the vestibular system and proprioception, which leads to simulator sickness. The frequency and severity of simulator sickness depends on the type of VR device (HMD vs. non-wearable displays), the type of tasks (e.g. walking vs. driving), and the users' clinical and demographical features

(ii) Other side effects:
Headache, dizziness, computer-related eye fatigue, reduced threshold of seizures, falls

Summary for the evidence for VR rehabilitation

VR rehabilitation has been found to be clinically useful in neurorehabilitation especially stroke, geriatric rehabilitation (e.g. falls, dementia), and musculoskeletal rehabilitation showing promise to complement pain management, oncological rehabilitation of breast cancer patients and balance rehabilitation for individuals suffering from spinal cord injury. It potentially creates a realistic environment for an individual to interact to perform intensive and repetitive exercises to maximise motor learning and neuroplasticity.

D. Brain computer interfaces in stroke rehabilitation

In the last decade, **brain computer interfaces (BCI)** have emerged as promising and useful tools for motor restoration employing motor imagery-induced EEG (electroencephalogram) to decode brain signals. However, to date, they remain as research tools for stroke rehabilitation, with a handful of commercially deployed BCI interfaces.

What are brain computer interfaces (BCI)?

In the context of motor rehabilitation for stroke, BCI systems decode patients' intent to move their paretic limbs through motor imagery EEG (MI-EEG) signals via externally applied scalp electrodes or internally implanted arrays. In doing so, they bypass injured motor segments in the brain and spinal cord, facilitating operation of a variety of end-effectors (e.g. robots, neuromuscular electrical stimulation, haptic feedback, or virtual imagery) without physical touch.

BCI systems can be divided into 2 main subtypes:

(i) **Assistive** BCI systems which aim to completely bypass the damaged neuronal pathways by providing alternative, continuous, and permanent control for communication and control of external devices (e.g. wheelchairs, keyboards, touchless communicators) for those with severe motor paralysis (e.g. locked in syndrome, high spinal cord injury)

(ii) **Rehabilitative** BCI systems which aim for recovery of damaged neuronal pathways through facilitation of neuroplasticity thereby restoring impaired motor functions

BCI, through bridging the intent of motor movement with sensori-motor feedback can result in measurable gains in motor function. To date, the largest field of BCI clinical applications with the most investigation involves that of post-stroke motor rehabilitation.

Neuroplasticity resulting from BCI intervention can be conceptualised through 4 broad mechanisms: (i) Neurofeedback training, (ii) Operant conditioning by reinforcement, (iii) Reinforcement of neuronal circuits by repetitive engagement and (iv) Hebbian learning ("neurons that fire together, wire together").

EEG-based BCI has a central role of neuro-feedback to self-regulate EEG activity which have may have multiple effects on motor, speech, cognitive functions (attention and memory) and mood via several mechanisms, i.e. upregulation of alpha waves or downregulation of beta, theta, and delta waves.

Brief summary of evidence for BCI for stroke rehabilitation

- A meta-analysis of BCI studies in 2018 observed that BCI intervention was associated with upper limb motor improvements, comparable with other widely used therapies including constraint-induced movement therapy, mirror therapy, and robotics[2]
- Regarding BCI and lower limb post stroke applications, preliminary studies have suggested possible benefits of BCI-functional electrical stimulation and visual imagery systems applied to the lower limb in randomised controlled trials, but challenges exist about the precise localisation of deep cortical foot and ankle areas; and distributed cortical areas compared to central pattern generator for gait activation

- With regards to the **non-motor effects** on EEG and BCI on unconscious states in the context of acquired brain injuries, recent reports indicate a dissociation between commanded behavioural abilities of patients to move their hands on command, compared to brain activation using EEG in 25% with better outcomes in those with the phenomenon of **cognitive motor dissociation**

- Potential applications for future: post stroke cognition. As MI-BCI systems require sustained visual attention span for extended amounts treatment of post stroke cognition manoeuvres

In conclusion, rehabilitation technology will continue to evolve rapidly in the depth of evidence and scope of clinical practice allowing rehabilitation professionals to strengthen both top-down and bottom-up approaches to achieve optimal outcomes for patients, at the same time allowing us to understand brain-behaviour relationships.

References

1. Chua KSG, Kuah CWK. Rehabilitation technology in the real world: promises, potentials, and perspectives. *Am J Phys Med Rehabil* 2017;96:S150–S156.

2. Bodien YG, Allanson J, Cardone P, Bonhomme A, Carmona J, Chatelle C, Chennu S, Conte M, Dehaene S, Finoia P, Heinonen G, Hersh JE, Kamau E, Lawrence PK, Lupson VC, Meydan A, Rohaut B, Sanders WR, Sitt JD, Soddu A, Valente M, Velazquez A, Voss HU, Vrosgou A, Claassen J, Edlow BL, Fins JJ, Gosseries O, Laureys S, Menon D, Naccache L, Owen AM, Pickard J, Stamatakis EA, Thibaut A, Victor JD, Giacino JT, Bagiella E, Schiff ND. Cognitive motor dissociation in disorders of consciousness. *N Engl J Med* 2024 Aug 15;391(7):598–608. doi: 10.1056/NEJMoa2400645. PMID: 39141852.

16

Sex and Sexuality in the Disabled

TOH Ee Mui Shirlene, LUI Wen Li, CHAN Wai Lim William

Albert is a 36-year-old gentleman who sustained a spinal cord injury with tetraplegia after a road traffic accident 6 months ago. He is recently married and is ready to start a family. He has erectile dysfunction and is unable to ejaculate. He uses vacuum constriction device and can achieve erection for intercourse. However, his sexual activity is intermittently affected by headache associated with high BP of 180/100 mmHg which disappears with cessation of sexual activity.

Introduction

- The World Health Organization definition of sexual health: sexual health is the state of physical, emotional, mental, and social well-being in relation to sexuality; it is not merely the absence of disease, dysfunction, or infirmity. Sexual health requires a positive and respectful approach to sexuality and sexual relationships, as well as the possibility of having pleasurable and safe sexual experiences, free of coercion, discrimination, and violence
- There is an inherent human yearning for intimacy, companionship, and physical satisfaction that sexuality affords
- However, disability often has a negative impact on sexual functioning

Sexual dysfunction after a disability

- Types of sexual dysfunction (DSM-5)
    - Male sexual dysfunctions
        - Male hypoactive sexual desire disorder
        - Premature ejaculation
        - Delayed ejaculation
        - Erectile disorder

- Female sexual dysfunction
  - Female sexual interest/arousal disorder
  - Female orgasmic disorder
  - Genito-pelvic pain/penetration disorder
- Other dysfunction
  - Substance/medication-induced sexual dysfunction
  - Other specified sexual dysfunction
  - Unspecified sexual dysfunction

Sexual dysfunction after disability may be due to

- Primary physical changes
  - Altered genital sensation
  - Decreased vaginal lubrication
  - Erectile dysfunction
  - Delayed ejaculation
  - Anorgasmia
- Secondary physical limitations (makes sexual activity unpleasant or challenging)
  - Fatigue
  - Pain
  - Motor deficits (e.g. weakness)
  - Spasticity and contractures
  - Bowel and bladder dysfunction
  - Cognitive impairment
- Psychosocial contributions
  - Poor self-esteem and body image issues
  - Anxiety and depression
- Effect of comorbid conditions
  - Diabetes, cardiovascular disease
- Medication-related factors
  - Medications prescribed can lead to sexual dysfunction

Sexual dysfunction in individuals with spinal cord injury (SCI)

- Sexual dysfunction after SCI is common
    - Erectile dysfunction
        - In individuals with complete upper motor neurone lesions above the conus (S2-4)
            - Unable to achieve psychogenic erections
            - Reflex erections (often unpredictable and limited) are preserved
        - In individuals with complete lower motor neurone lesions
            - Psychogenic erections poorly sustained
            - Unable to achieve reflex erections
    - Delayed ejaculation/anejaculation
    - Loss of genital sensation
    - Decreased vaginal lubrication
    - Decreased arousal and orgasm
- Physical effects and complications of SCI make sexual activity challenging
    - Paralysis — affects positioning and movement
    - Pain
    - Neurogenic bladder and bowel
    - Spasticity
    - Autonomic dysreflexia — a medical emergency and can be precipitated by sexual stimulation
    - Pressure injury

Sexual dysfunction in individuals with stroke and traumatic brain injury

- Sexual dysfunction is common after stroke and traumatic brain injury (TBI)
    - Erectile and ejaculatory dysfunction (40–50% in males)
    - Decreased sexual drive (20–50%)
    - Decreased vaginal lubrication (50% in females)
    - Decreased orgasm

- Decreased sexual satisfaction
- Hypersexual behaviour can occur after TBI

- Physical effects of stroke make sexual activity challenging
  - Hemiparesis: affects positioning and movement
  - Neglect
  - Visual field defects
  - Neurogenic bladder and bowel
  - Spasticity

Sexual dysfunction in individuals with limb amputation

- Usually have preserved sexual genital functioning
- Physical effects of amputation make sexual activity challenging
  - Impaired balance and movement → difficulty with body positioning
  - Phantom sensation and pain

Sexual dysfunction related to medication use

- If sexual dysfunction occurs as a result of a medication, it is often necessary to switch to a different class of medication
- Alternatively, in men, medications like a phosphodiesterase-5 (PDE-5) inhibitor can be used to counteract the sexual side effects of medications
- Medications commonly used in rehabilitation that may cause sexual dysfunction include anti-hypertensives (alpha and beta blockers), anti-depressants (selective serotonin reuptake inhibitors and serotonin-norepinephrine reuptake inhibitors), antipsychotics (ripserdal, quetiapine), anti-spasticity medications (baclofen, benzodiazepines), neurostimulants (methylphenidate and amantadine may cause hypersexual behaviour), and medications for treating neuropathic pain (gabapentin, pregabalin)

Assessment of an individual with sexual dysfunction after a disability

- Use PLISSIT model to facilitate conversation
  - The PLISSIT model was developed by Annon as a framework for care providers to assist in the ordering and treatment of sexual problems. The model consists of four steps for addressing sexual

concerns: **Permission, Limited information, Specific suggestions and Intensive therapy**

- **Permission:** the provider creates the space for a patient to bring up sexual health concerns, usually through open ended questions such as "Is there anything about your sexual health you'd like to discuss?" or "Individual with spinal cord injury may experience issue with their relationship, do you have any concerns?"
- **Limited information:** once the patient has identified a concern, the provider can provide relevant information to address this concern. This can include dispelling myth and providing facts on potential causes of the symptoms
- **Specific suggestions:** a differential diagnosis is offered, with specific suggestions on how to begin addressing the problem. The provider will usually discuss with the patient on the possible recommendations and engage the patient/couple to prioritise the recommendations
- **Intensive therapy:** if necessary, a referral can be made to a sexual health specialist, such as a sex therapist, pelvic floor specialist, or sex educator, to provide more comprehensive support and guidance

- History
  - Type of sexual dysfunction: decreased sexual desire, erectile dysfunction, ejaculatory dysfunction, pain, decreased vaginal lubrication, orgasmic dysfunction, decreased genital sensation
  - Medical history and surgical history
    - Cardiovascular disease
    - Hypertension, hyperlipidaemia, diabetes
    - Malignancy, benign prostatic hypertrophy
    - Endocrine disorder
    - Neurological disorder (spinal cord injury/traumatic brain injury/stroke)
  - Medication history
  - Substance use: smoking, alcohol, recreational drug use
  - Reproductive history, gynaecological history, menstrual history
  - Sexual history: sexual practices, number and gender of partners, history of sexually transmitted diseases, birth control method
  - Psychosocial history: depression, anxiety, life stressors, relationship dynamics

- Physical examination
    - Physical impairments
        - Motor and sensory examination
        - Limb loss
        - Range of motion of joints
        - Spasticity
        - Balance
    - Functional status
    - Genital examination
- Investigations — to be done as necessary to rule out causes of sexual dysfunction

Non-pharmacological management

- Open communication between the couple to address issues of role change/reversal and attitudes towards sexuality and intimacy is important. Below are some tips for better communication:
    - Be honest to share any insecurities or anxieties. Focus on the current situation and support each other's vulnerabilities
    - Be personal by expressing one's own needs from a personal perspective. Talk from the first person using the words "I" and "My" instead of "You" statements
    - Pay attention to each other's verbal and non-verbal responses. Be sensitive to each other's reactions and pace the conversation accordingly
    - Focus on responding and not be reactive. A reactive mode of communication is often based on past experiences may seem as being defensive
    - Make a request and not a complaint. By converting a complaint into a specific action request, this will help the partner focus on the present situation and prevent any previous unresolved conflicts from surfacing
- Changes in sensation
    - Emphasise stimulation of unaffected body parts
    - Explore new erogenous zones (areas sensitive to touch include lips, neck, inner of the thighs) with different strokes

- Muscle weakness and muscle stiffness
    - If the upper limbs are affected, consider the use aids (vibrators) for stimulation
    - Use of momentum (rocking in a waterbed can help with movement)
    - Consider the use of pillow/wedge for support
    - Explore use of assistive device such as hoist and wheelchair
- Muscle spasm
    - Gentle stretching of the affected muscles can easily be incorporated into foreplay
    - Try to explore positions that inhibit spasms accordingly
- Urinary/bowel incontinence
    - Discuss about the possibility of a bladder or bowel accident to avoid surprises and to ease anxiety
    - Limit fluid intake prior to intercourse and to empty the bladder/ bowel prior to sexual activity
    - Keep towels/urinal nearby and protect the mattress with waterproof bedsheet or underpad if possible
- Feeling of fatigue/tired
    - Find positions that require less physical exertion or take a less active role in sexual activity
    - Consider use sex aids or toys for sexual arousal
    - Explore alternative activities for intimacy such as caressing and kissing
- Lack of vaginal lubrication
    - Use water based lubricants
    - Take time to enjoy the sense of touch and communicate with each other. Do not rush into an intercourse
    - Incorporate relaxation techniques such as massage and heat therapy as part of foreplay
- Changes in body image
    - Medical equipment such as prosthesis and wheelchairs, body brace, and other adaptive equipment are incorporated as part of the patient body image

- The altered physical appearance will result in patient's feeling of unattractiveness and having a negative opinion of their own personal value and sexual desirability
  - Keeping a positive self-image by maintaining a neat and fresh look with good personal hygiene

Pharmacological management for erectile dysfunction

- Erectile dysfunction
  - Non-pharmacological
    - Vacuum constriction device — applies a negative pressure to draw blood into corpora cavernosa which is then retained by the application of a constriction band at the base of the penis
      - Pros: high efficacy rate (90%)
      - Cons: unnatural appearance of erection, penile pain, trapped ejaculate
      - Constriction band contraindicated in those with severe bleeding disorder (anticoagulant therapy is a relative contraindication), priapism, or severe penile curvature
      - Constriction band should not be left in place for more than half an hour due to risk of ischemia (especially in individuals with SCI who may be insensate)
  - Pharmacological
    - Oral PDE5 (phosphodiesterase 5) inhibitors
      - Side effects: headache, flushing, rhinitis, back pain, hearing loss
      - Contraindicated with use of nitrates
    - Intraurethral alprostadil
    - Intracavernosal injection
      - Cons: requires training, high discontinuation rate due to penile pain, priapism
  - Surgical
    - Penile prosthesis

Conclusion

Albert and his wife underwent sexuality counselling and learnt how to better communicate with each other. This allowed them to understand each other's perspectives and needs. His symptom of headache associated with high blood pressure during sexual activity was assessed to be a result of autonomic dysreflexia (a condition unique to patients with spinal cord injury)* due to improper positioning and bladder distension. Apart from adopting a suitable and comfortable position, he was advised to empty his bladder and bowel prior to sexual activity. The couple later successfully conceived with assisted reproductive technology.

*For more details on autonomic dysreflexia, please refer to the chapter on "Spinal Cord Injury Rehabilitation".

17

A Holistic Approach to Return to Work and Driving After a Disability

SETIOTA Nuez Odessa, SOH Yan Ming,
CHAN Mei Leng, LIM Hui Hui

Return to work

The value of work to one's health and well-being is well-documented. It contributes to one's financial security and is also closely tied to one's self-identity and sense of purpose and belonging. Work participation has been shown to promote physical and mental health and recovery. It is also associated with better life satisfaction in individuals with disabilities. In fact, returning to gainful employment is an important mark of successful rehabilitation.

Understanding the demands and capacity for returning to work

Returning to the workplace after recovering from an acute illness is something that almost every working adult has experienced with little consequence or worry for the nearby future.

However, for persons living with a debilitating/chronic health condition or an acquired disability, successfully returning to work can be a huge barrier to overcome. Even if one is able to successfully return to work, staying on the job remains a constant challenge that these individuals face. It often entails a process of personal adjustment and learning about their own strengths, coping with their functional limitations and condition-related symptoms, and managing their expectations of their recovery process.

The ability of an individual to carry out job functions is dependent on the interaction between his/her capacities, the job and task characteristics and work demands, and the physical and social environment in which he/she is performing the job. A structured and multifaceted approach can then be taken for intervention planning.

In stroke patients, problems faced when returning to work include oversensitivity to external stimuli (noise or lights), difficulty resuming tasks if interrupted, requiring a longer time to process information and instructions or difficulty remembering details.[1] There are impairments that are 'invisible' and may not be readily understood by the healthcare professional, employer, co-workers, or even patients themselves. The most important invisible impairment causing difficulties at work is fatigue. Patients may not be aware of stroke-related fatigue which affects work productivity. This can lead to overestimation of one's own abilities with the patient returning to pre-morbid workload and duties prematurely.

Similarly, cancer survivors have reported fatigue and cognitive difficulties, and other cancer treatment-related symptoms (e.g. blurry vision, nausea, neuropathy) as impediments to work functioning. They often struggle with emotional distress, undesired changes to their appearance and the need to juggle between work and treatment commitments.[2]

The return-to-work process is complex and involves numerous stakeholders with different expertise, responsibilities, and objectives. Thus, individuals looking to return to work often benefit from help with navigating resources and returning to the workplace in a phased manner. A graded return to work plan and a conducive workplace for thriving at work can be built through effective coordination between healthcare professionals, a well-informed employer, and supportive co-workers.

Role of physicians

Getting help and support from the patient's primary care physician is necessary for their return-to-work endeavours. Firstly, physicians can adopt a biopsychosocial approach towards recovery and work disability. This involves making an effort to explore and address patients' attitudes, beliefs, and possible contextual and psychosocial barriers to their recovery and work rehabilitation.[3]

Secondly, physicians can help patients to shift away from the misconception that "full recovery" or "eradication of impairments" needs to be achieved before they are able to return to work. This can be done through proper education on prognostication and refocusing on identifying suitable duties by matching their current abilities with their work demands. This supports realistic expectations and goal setting for an earlier return to work.

Lastly, while physicians serve as gatekeepers to ensure fitness for work resumption through the issuance of sick leave, they are also encouraged to consider the provision of "fit notes" with specific instructions on the patient's functional abilities and restrictions to their employers. This is critical to allow arrangements for necessary accommodations, such as reducing working hours or restructuring the job scope, that would aid enhanced adjustment and coping post transition to work.

Services are available within the healthcare and social service sectors in Singapore to support persons with disability in the return to gainful employment. Physicians also play a pivotal role in facilitating timely and appropriate access to these services to aid work reintegration. Where relevant, various allied health services can be enlisted to aid in assessment and objective determination of work readiness. These professionals also train patients in the use of strategies (e.g. external memory aids, pacing, relaxation techniques, work simplification) and assistive technology (e.g. use of smartphones, modified keyboard, or voice recognition software), and provide employers with recommendations and access to resources for workplace modification and adjustments to optimise work functions. Occupational therapists, or return-to-work coordinators in some institutions, can also facilitate the implementation of a person-centred return to work plan via communication with and coordination of the different stakeholders.

Planning for return to work involves coordination between the employer, primary care physician, occupational therapist, physiotherapist, and if needed, the psychologist, medical social worker, and speech therapist, in order to understand the visible and invisible problems after any illness with residual physical, cognitive, or psychological difficulties. Proper coordination supports a better transition back into the workplace and improves the chances of successfully returning to and staying in the job.

Physicians and occupational health practitioners and therapists should also take into account other barriers that may indirectly affect returning to work successfully, such as not being able to drive, inadequate financial resources or lack of benefits.

Factors affecting return-to-work outcomes

Irrespective of nature and type of disability, the following factors influence return-to-work outcomes:

1. Employer support and work accommodations

Employer support affects the chances of successfully returning to work. Support can range from providing adequate sick leave, modifying the job scope or the work schedule. Early engagement and communication with the different stakeholders, i.e. the employer, occupational therapist, primary healthcare physician or specialist is associated with a positive return to work outcome. Centralizing the case management, through a multidisciplinary team approach in collaboration with the workplace improves outcomes on return to work. Work accommodations, such as a modified job scope or graduated work exposure with onsite work evaluation, can be applied across different health conditions and is an important factor for improving return to work outcomes. Delays in returning to work were reduced if the interventions included early contact with the employer or workplace by the healthcare provider, work accommodation offers, doing worksite visits, and the presence of a return-to-work coordinator.

2. Educational level and income status

Patients who had higher educational qualifications and/or held professional or managerial jobs were more likely to return to work. Higher income earners were more likely to return to work compared to those with lower income. Those with higher educational attainment or managerial careers have improved return to work outcomes and is related to the perceived value of skill sets, and thus better employment assistance. Patients with higher self-efficacy and optimistic expectations of recovery and return to work were more likely to have positive return-to-work outcomes.

In patients with a stroke or brain injury, cognition is the most consistent negative predictor of return to work. Problems in doing more complex tasks, concentration, working memory and processing speed also have a negative impact on high level jobs or tasks. For some patients, detailed neuropsychological assessment may be needed to gain more insight into the cognitive strengths and weaknesses to provide the necessary interventions and ensure successful reintegration into the workplace.

Domains for return-to-work interventions

To provide emphasis in providing a multipronged approach in helping patients successfully return to work, Cullen *et al.*,[4] has described it into several interventions.

1. Health focused interventions — this includes medical assessment, graded activity and exercise, work hardening, cognitive behavioural therapy through a multidisciplinary team approach i.e. physical therapy, occupational therapy, and psychological therapy
2. Service coordination interventions — initiation of communication between the healthcare providers and the workplace is essential with the main aim of improving delivery and access to return-to-work services involving the workplace. This includes development of return-to-work planning, education and training and case management
3. Work modification interventions — this involves modifying work conditions, examples of which are provision of modified duties, modified working hours, supernumerary replacements, ergonomic adjustments, or other worksite adjustments
4. Multi-domain interventions — this is a combination of at least two of the three intervention domains. There is strong evidence that multiple domain

interventions are effective in improving return to work outcomes in workers with musculoskeletal, pain-related, or mental health conditions. This aligned with one of the dominant theoretical paradigms in the work disability and return to work literature, the Sherbrooke model. This model proposes that multidisciplinary and multi-factorial interventions that seek to address an array of individual and societal factors that influence return to work are likely to be effective

Case Illustrations

Case 1

A 50-year-old female, married, working as a secondary school teacher, was admitted in the orthopedics ward after sustaining a lumbar spinal cord injury. She developed paraplegia and urinary incontinence. After 6 weeks of inpatient physiotherapy and occupational therapy, she was discharged back home. She is unable to stand or ambulate due to the severity of the weakness of her lower limbs. However, she was able to independently transfer from her bed to a wheelchair and self-propel her wheelchair within her own home environment. She is independent in doing her self-care activities, such as dressing and showering. She is able to independently do intermittent catheterization every 6 hours as part of her urinary bladder care.

She has contacted her school principal/supervisor that she will be on medical leave as she still needs to undergo outpatient rehabilitation and that she intends to return to work once she is able to.

As part of a multidisciplinary team approach, the planning for return to work was centralized through a case manager, working in collaboration with the different stakeholders, i.e. school principal/supervisor, occupational and physical therapist, rehabilitation medicine physician.

To illustrate further, in this scenario, the health focused interventions include graded activity or exercise, a work hardening individualised program, through regular physical and occupational therapy, and medical assessments.

She requires medical assessments to ensure that she is able to manage her urinary bladder and bowel care with the aim of avoiding urinary and bowel accidents when she's outside of her home or eventually when she's in the workplace. This includes advice on fluid intake or fluid restriction, monitoring urine volumes during self-catheterization and monitoring for any urinary leakage or incontinence. She temporarily needs to wear incontinence pads when she intends to go out in the community. She also needs to take medications, such as laxatives, or advise on the type of dietary intake to regulate her bowel clearance with the aim of preventing bowel accidents when out in the community.

Planning for return to work also requires training to be independent in wheelchair mobility in the community, including independence in taking public transport such as taking the bus or train. This includes training in the use of a motorized wheelchair.

Under the domains of service coordination and work modification interventions, the occupational therapist concurrently coordinates with the employer to plan on eventual return to work with some modification of working conditions, such as altering job duties and modifying working hours. Early communication with the school principal/supervisor or work colleagues enables more awareness of the patient's capacity and enabling factors for successfully returning to work. Other work modification interventions include ensuring wheelchair accessibility to and within the workplace (e.g. ramp installation). The occupational therapist would also need to coordinate with the workplace supervisor to ensure wheelchair accessibility to the nearest washroom for the patient to do intermittent catheterization timely.

The primary physician ensures that the patient is covered with sufficient medical leave. Based on the patient's progress or readiness to return to work and the multidisciplinary team assessment, the primary physician will need to recommend to the employer the need for any modification of job duties or gradual exposure back to work such as starting with reduced working hours, until the patient is able to return to full time duties.

The patient is also on follow up with the psychologist to provide emotional support and counselling as the patient was assessed to have low mood issues which may affect her participation during therapy and possibly, return to work.

Amongst all the coordination and communication efforts with the different stakeholders and the employer, the patient's consent and motivation must be taken into account. Hence, communication with the patient on her own goals and readiness on returning to work must also considered.

The patient was able to return to teaching with modified working hours in the beginning, i.e. thrice a week, 4 hours each time. Her worksite was modified to allow wheelchair accessibility and a ramp was installed for her to be able to access the nearest washroom. Regular communication with the school principal/supervisor was needed to prepare the patient to return to full time work.

Multi-domain interventions with a multidisciplinary team approach thus helps patients to successfully return to work.

Case 2

A 62-year-old male, widower, working as an office cleaner, was admitted for a mild stroke. It affected his ability to ambulate independently and ability to perform his basic self-care activities, such as dressing, showering and toileting. He requires minimal assistance to ambulate short distances within the home environment, plus a walking frame as a mobility aid. The patient does not have any cognitive impairments or any mood issues after the stroke. He was very keen to be able to return to work.

The patient has already initiated informing his employer of his stroke condition, the need for continued rehabilitation with the aim of returning to work. The employer was very forthcoming and the human resource officer-in-charge contacted the rehabilitation team early to inquire on the length of medical leave necessary and the readiness of the patient to return to work. The patient was allowed by his employer to take prolonged medical leave as recommended by his doctor to undergo post-stroke rehabilitation with the aim of returning to work.

The multi-domain interventions include continued physical and occupational therapy, including an individualised work hardening program. The medical social worker provides assistance for outpatient services where financial constraints are identified. As the patient improves, the case manager or occupational therapist will coordinate with the employer and plan for gradual re-exposure to work or modify working hours and job duties. The physiotherapist will need to assess if the patient is able to access public transport independently when going to and back from work. The occupational therapist may recommend modifying work hours at the initial phase of returning to work, for instance, starting with 4 hours a day of work, 3 times a week. The multidisciplinary team and employer need constant communication in reviewing the patient's readiness to return to his full-time job or previous job responsibilities, taking into consideration the patient's own goals and receptiveness on returning to work.

Return to driving

Returning to driving is an important aspect of one's life that can significantly be affected after an injury or medical condition with resulting physical or cognitive impairments. It affects the ability to resume one's occupation, accessibility to and from one's work site or limit one's ability to continue recreational or leisure activities.

Driving is a complex task that can be affected by cognitive, motor, visual and perceptual deficits. As the primary physician, making a thorough medical assessment for patients who would want to return to driving is warranted. In addition, the primary physician should also discuss with the patient the intention for the need to return to driving, whether for vocational, personal, or recreational purposes.

As there is paucity in evidence-based screening tools for assessing fitness to drive, a combination of approaches can be used by primary care physicians. An example is the SAFE DRIVE checklist.[5] These include:

Safety record — history of driving problems

Attention skills — look for lapses of consciousness or recurrent episodes of confusion

Family report — ask family members about observations of driving ability

Ethanol — screen for alcohol abuse

Drugs — conduct a medication review, checking for sedating or anticholinergic drugs

Reaction time — check for neurologic or musculoskeletal disorders that could slow reactions

Intellectual impairment — conduct a mini-mental state examination

Vision and visuospatial function — test for visual acuity

Executive function — check ability to plan and sequence activities and self-monitor behaviours

If there are any concerns noted in any of these areas, referral to a specialized centre is recommended.

In stroke patients, cognitive and motor impairments are negative predictors of return to driving. Cognitive impairments of visuospatial abilities, attention, problem solving, and organizational capabilities, are important predictors of driving as driving requires a response to the multiple complex demands of driving and traffic demand. Other factors to be considered in assessing patient's fitness to drive are premorbid driving history i.e. personality and risk-taking behaviours pre-injury. Patients post brain injury may have reduced self-awareness and lack of insight into deficits and may rate themselves as having excellent driving skills.

After the medical practitioner does the screening and clinical assessment, if suitable, a referral is made to the driver assessor occupational therapist to do an off-road assessment. For off-road assessments, fitness to drive generally includes testing for visual function, cognition, and physical impairments. As driving is a highly complex visual task, clinical assessment for vision does not only include testing for visual acuity but is supplemented with tests for visual field, visual inattention, visual processing speed, and scanning. Assessment for cognitive functioning mainly includes testing for 4 domains, i.e. attention, executive function, visual spatial, and visual perceptual skills. Assessment for physical impairments includes range of motion, motor strength, muscle tone, coordination, balance, proprioception, and mobility.

For patients who have spinal cord injury (SCI), paraplegia, lower extremity amputations or impairments, assessments for fitness to drive can be more challenging as patients will need to train on driving skills with the use of car adaptations, the use of hand controls, and/or prosthesis. This needs learning of new motor and cognitive skills to ensure safety in driving. For patients with spinal cord injury, patients need to balance driving in response to environmental demands such as vibration and still able to maintain a well-supported seating position while operating a vehicle with car adaptations.

After the off-road assessment, if suitable, the driver assessor occupational therapist proceeds to do an on-road assessment. The on-road assessment is still the typical gold standard for assessing medical fitness to drive.

The Singapore Medical Association (SMA) has guidelines, for medical practitioners to assess patients' medical fitness to drive. Familiarity with the guidelines is important to manage expectations for patients who intend to return to driving. To illustrate, Table 1 shows the guidelines for assessment of medical fitness to drive for post stroke patients.[6]

Table 1. Summary on the SMA guidelines for stroke (2nd edition).

	Group 1 (class 1,2 and 3 licenses)	Group 2 (class 4,5 and vocational licenses)
Stroke	Patients without any residual disability may resume driving after 1 month Patients with disabilities such as residual weakness, significant visual field defects, perceptual or mental impairment, incoordination, etc. severe enough to interfere with control of the vehicle should not drive Patients with mild residual disabilities that may not interfere with control of the vehicle may undergo DARP* > 1 month after stroke. They may be allowed to drive if they pass DARP*, after final review by a neurologist	Able to return to driving if all of the following conditions are met: • > 1 year post stroke • Stroke is not due to high-risk underlying condition which is left untreated (e.g. high grade carotid stenosis, untreated aneurysm) • Fully recovered • Passed DARP* • Compliant with treatment • Final clearance given by a neurologist

*DARP — Driving Assessment and Rehabilitation Programme

There could be changes to the SMA guidelines at intervals i.e. currently only the 2nd edition is available, but a 3rd edition has been planned with changes to some sections, including the 1-year delay for taxi drivers post stroke (there is intention of making it shorter following feedback from the medical fraternity).

Driving assessment and rehabilitation programs in Singapore

In the Singapore setting, primary care physicians can refer to driving rehabilitation specialists to further evaluate patients with medical conditions, especially those with resulting physical or cognitive changes that precludes safety in driving.

The institutions offering these programs are 1) Driving Assessment and Rehabilitation Programme (DARP) in Tan Tock Seng Hospital, 2) Driving Assessment and Rehabilitation Service (DARS) in JurongHealth, Ng Teng Fong General Hospital and Jurong Community Hospital and 3) SGH Driving Evaluation and Rehabilitation Service (SGH DrivERS) in SingHealth, Singapore General Hospital, and Outram Community Hospital. The occupational therapist in these programs specialises in assessing a client's ability to return to driving safely with reference to the Medical Guidelines on Fitness to Drive (Singapore Medical Association, 2011) and the requirements of the Traffic Police (Road Traffic Act).

The occupational therapist will do a comprehensive driving assessment which starts with the off-road assessment. The medical history, previous driving history, visual, physical, and cognitive functioning are assessed. The off-road evaluation helps to anticipate any difficulties in the on-road component of the evaluation.

If suitable, patients would proceed to do an on-road assessment. If needed, the therapist will recommend and arrange for the appropriate vehicle modifications (Table 2). The occupational therapist may also arrange for specialized driving rehabilitation and refresher lessons with qualified driving instructors, i.e. from the Handicap Welfare Association (HWA) to help patients return to driving. All final reports from DARP, DARS, and SGH DrivERS need to be endorsed by the referring doctor, to certify full medical fitness to drive.

Table 2. Commonly used adaptive driving equipment.

Device	Purpose
Hand controls	Enables acceleration and braking for drivers with lower limb limitations (e.g. push/pull, push/right angle pull, push/twist, power assisted control units)
Left foot acceleration	For drivers with impairment in the right lower extremity
Steering assistive devices	Allows access to all steering requirements with one extremity (e.g. spinner knobs, bi-pins, tri-pins)

The car park label scheme supports persons with mobility impairment who require vehicular transportation. A valid label permits parking in designated accessible parking lots that allow driver and/or passengers with mobility impairment to fully open the vehicle doors to board or alight.

Case Illustration

Case 1

A 44-year-old male, working as a project manager, was discharged from hospital after a stroke 8 weeks ago. He underwent inpatient rehabilitation in a community hospital setting and had good functional recovery. He was assessed to be independent in community ambulation and self-care activities.

Before the stroke, he drives his personal car to work and holds a valid driving class 3 license. As a project manager, he needs to meet clients in different sites and to supervise other employees in his team.

Upon follow up with his primary care physician, he enquired if he could return to driving. He enjoys driving for leisure activities and helps him continue to do his work more efficiently.

Upon assessment by his primary care physician, he still has residual right sided upper limb weakness with limited right shoulder range of motion. There are no cognitive or visual impairments. A referral was made to DARP for further assessment for fitness to drive.

The patient passed both DARP off-road and on-road assessments for a class 3 driving license with a recommendation for a spinner knob. The referring doctor endorses the recommendations from DARP and certifies the patient as medically fit to drive.

References

1. Scott SL, Burns SP *et al.* Returning to work after mild stroke. *Archives of Physical Medicine and Rehabilitation.* 2019;100(2):379–383.

2. Sun WJ, Chen K *et al.* Work-related barriers, facilitators, and strategies of breast cancer survivors working during curative treatment. *Work.* 2016;55(4):783–795.

3. See B, Chia SE *et al.* Return to work is an important therapeutic goal. *Ann Acad Med Singap.* 2017;46(6):245–247.

4. Cullen KL, Irvin E *et al.* Effectiveness of workplace interventions in return-to-work for musculoskeletal, pain-related and mental health conditions:

an update of the evidence and messages for practitioners. *J Occup Rehabil.* 2017;28(1):1–15.

5. Molnar FJ, Byszewski AM *et al.* In-office evaluation of medical fitness to drive: practical approaches for assessing older people. *Can Fam Physician.* 2005;51(3):372–379.

6. *Singapore medical association medical guidelines on fitness to drive*, 2nd edition. (2011).

Index

Alternative and Augmentative
  Communication (AAC), 173–175
anterior cruciate ligament (ACL) injury,
  145
acquired communication disorders
  assessment, 172
  rehabilitation, 173
adrenocortiotropic hormone (ACTH)
  deficiency, 40
acute agitation escalation, 37
adaptive control, and progression, 216
adaptive driving equipment, 244
anti-diuretic hormone (ADH)
  deficiency, 40
advanced age, 34
aerobic exercise, 115
algometer, 129
allodynia, 126
anatomical hand arches, 203
angina, 116
ankle foot dynamic synergy, 206
ankle support, 146
antalgic gait, 140
anterior drawer test, 146
anterior knee pain, 143
Anticares, 218
anxiety, 115
aortic stenosis, 116
aphasia, 171
  assessment, 172
  drugs and treatment of, 177
  recovery, 176
  type of, 172
approach, 219
apraxia, 18
areflexic bowel, 52, 67, 69
arthritis, 117
assistive technology, 237
attention, working memory, 45
autonomic dysreflexia, 54, 60, 62, 64–66,
  227, 233
autonomic function, 38

basal skull, facial, 40
blood pressures, 117
botulinum toxin, 189
brain computer interfaces (BCI), 213, 221
breathlessness, 115, 123
  techniques, 121
button hook, 192

cancer associated cognitive dysfunction,
  93
cancer-related fatigue, 88, 89
  brief fatigue inventory, 88
  energy conservation techniques, 90
  EORTC QLQ-C30, 88
  nonpharmacological interventions, 90
  nutritional assessment, 89
  pharmacological agents, 90
car adaptations, 243
cardiac devices, 123
cardiovascular, 115
car park label scheme, 245
case management, 237
  service coordination, 240
  service coordination interventions, 238
cervicogenic dizziness, 134
cervicogenic headache, 133
chemotherapy induced peripheral
  neuropathy, 91
  coasting phenomenon, 91
  electrodiagnostic studies, 91
  exercise, 93
chronic ankle pain, 146
Clarke sign, 144
closed kinetic chain exercises, 145
cock-up splint, 203

cognitive, 238
  computer-aided rehabilitation, 45
  difficulties, 236
  disability, 42
  impairment, 117
  motor dissociation, 223
comorbidities, 33
compensating for impaired functions, 44
compensatory memory strategies, 42
confusion, disorientation, and agitation, 32
congestive heart failure, 116
contraindications to cardiopulmonary exercise, 116
chronic obstructive pulmonary disease (COPD), 121
core muscle function, 130

deconditioned, 11
deconditioning, 2, 4, 123
delirium subtype, 35
depression, 115
diabetes mellitus, 117
diffuse axonal injury (DAI), 34
disorders of consciousness (DOC), 47
double crush syndrome, 133
driver assessor occupational therapist, 242
driving assessment and rehabilitation programs, 244
dysarthria, types of, 171
dysphagia, 18, 24
  common causes, 165
  compensatory strategies, 168
  imaging assessment, 167
dysphasia, 17, 23, 29
dyspnea, 115
dysrhythmia, 117

post-traumatic seizures (PTS)
  early, 39
  late, 39
educational level, 238
  higher educational qualifications, 238
employer support, 237
endurance, 117, 121, 123
energy conservation strategies, 115
environmental modifications, 44
erectile dysfunction, 225–227, 229, 232
evidence-based approaches, 45
excessive stimulation, 35
exercise and safety concerns in cancer rehabilitation
  assessment of balance and mobility, 98, 99
exercise and safety concerns in cancer rehabilitation, 98
exercise prescription, 116
  frequency, 121, 123
  intensity, 121, 123
  time, 121, 123
  type, 121, 123

Flexion Abduction External Rotation (FABER), 140
falls and road accidents, 31
fatigue, 115, 123, 236
fitness
  for work, 236
  to drive, 242, 243
FITT
  Frequency, 117
  Intensity, 117
  Time, 117
  Type, 117
FITT principle, 117
flexible endoscopic evaluation of swallowing, 167
Foot Care and Limb Design Centre, 114
forearm gutter crutch, 196
formal neuropsychological assessment, 34
fractures, 117
frailty, 81
  syndrome, 79
functional decline, 2

gait, 106, 110, 111, 113
  patterns, 201
general measures of functional outcome, 42
genu recurvatum, 208
geriatric rehabilitation, 76
Glasgow Outcome Scale-Extended (GOS-E), 33
Glasgow Outcome Scale (GOS), 33

greater trochanteric pain syndrome (GTPS), 141, 142
groin pain, 140
ground reaction force, 204

heart
  block, 117
  failure, 123
  rate, 117
heel strike, 206
hemiplegia, 17
hip
  osteoarthritis, 140
  precautions, 141
  replacement, 141
hyperalgesia, 126

ICU-acquired weakness (ICUAW), 150, 151
ICU delirium, 153
iliotibial band syndrome (ITBS), 142, 143
immobilisation, 6
immobility, 2, 4
income status, 238
  higher income earners, 238
inhaler technique and compliance, 121

JFK Coma Recovery Scale-revised (CRS-R), 48

Karvonen formula, 117

Lachman test, 145
lateral hip pain, 141
lateral knee pain, 142
locked in syndrome and akinetic mutism, 47
long handled reacher, 192
lymphedema in cancer, 95

McConnell taping, 144
medical fitness to drive, 243
medicare functional level, 107
minimally conscious states (MCS), 47
misdiagnosis, 48
Modified Ashworth scale, 179, 183
Modified Barium, 167
Modified Borg Dyspnea Scale, 119
Montreal Cognitive Assessment, 34
motor imagery EEG (MI-EEG), 221
multi-domain interventions, 238, 241
muscle dysfunction, 128
myocardial infarction, 116
myocarditis, 116

neural
  mobilization, 135
  tension, 131
neurogenic bowel dysfunction, 66
neurogenic lower urinary tract dysfunction (NLUTD), 59–61, 65
neurological deficits, 117
neuromodulation, 49
neuropathic pain, 125
neuropharmacological, 36
neuropsychological testing, 41
noble compression test, 142
nociceptive pain, 125
non-pharmacological, 36
normal physiology of swallowing, 165

Ober test, 143
assessment
  off-road, 242, 244
  on-road, 243, 244
orthobiologic intervention, 147
orthostatic BP, 117
outcome, 21
oxygen therapy, 123

pain, 117, 123
palliative rehabilitation, 87
patellar
  grind test, 144
  tracking disorder, 144
patellofemoral pain syndrome, 143
Patrick test, 140
pericarditis, 116
phantom limb pain, 112
post-intensive care syndrome (PICS), 149, 150

post-intensive care syndrome-family (PICS-F), 154
pivot shift test, 145
plateau, 41
platelet rich plasma, 147
PLISSIT model, 228
post-ICU rehabilitation, 162
post-traumatic amnesia (PTA), 31
  emerged from, 41
  duration, 34
  scales, 34
potentially reversible, 35
pressure injuries, 69, 70
preventative rehabilitation, 87
procedural memory, 32
prolotherapy, 147
pulmonary, 115
  embolism, 116
  hypertension, 116, 123

back and neck pain
  red flags, 128
  yellow flags, 129
reflexic bowel, 66–68
regain awareness, 49
rehabilitation, 17, 20–24
  restorative, 87
remediation, 43
removable rigid dressing (RRD), 109
returning to driving, 241
  predictor, 242
returning to work, 235–237
  graded plan, 236
  participation, 235
  planning, 237
  predictor, 238
reversible organic, 45
robot-aided therapy (RAT), 213
rocker mechanism, 207

solid ankle cushioned heel (SACH), 107
sacroiliac joint (SIJ) dysfunctions, 130
sarcopenia, 80
self-propulsion, 194
sensory stimulation programmes, 49
serial clinical examinations, 33
serially monitor, 45
sexual dysfunction, 225–228
SG Enable, 191
sick leave, 236, 237
Singapore Medical Association, 243
spasticity, 28, 65, 66, 69, 72, 179, 180, 185–187
spinal cord injury, 51, 53–56, 59, 61, 65, 72
splints, 187
stair climb, 201
strengthening, 117, 121, 123
stroke, 17, 19–21, 24–28
stroke-related fatigue, 236
stump shaping, 106
subarachnoid haemorrhage, intraventricular haemorrhage, 34
subclinical state, 39
subdural haemorrhage, 34
supportive rehabilitation, 87
Surestep, 205
swallow study, 167

talar tilt test, 146
talk test, 119
Tardieu scale, 183, 184
target heart rate, 117
target specific neurocognitive problems, 45
telepractice, 175
tenodesis, 203
tilt-in-space wheelchair, 195
traumatic brain injury (TBI), 31
  3-6 month's post-TBI, 41
  inpatient rehabilitation programme, 32
  penetrating, 39

universal cuff, 192
unresponsive wakefulness syndrome, 47
urinary tract infection, 54, 55, 60, 61, 65

venous thromboembolism, 56
verticalization, 48
videofluroscopy swallow study, 167
virtual reality (VR) applications, 213, 219
VR-based technology (VRT), 219

Waddell signs, 134
wearable robotic exoskeletons, 215
wearable soft robotics, 218
work accommodations, 237
  graduated work exposure, 237
  modified job scope, 237
  onsite work evaluation, 237
  modification interventions, 238
workplace modification, 237
work rehabilitation, 236
  health focused interventions, 238
  work readiness, 237